Penguin Books

The Fabric of Mind

Richard Bergland was born in 1932 in Malta, Montana.
A graduate of Cornell Medical School in 1958, he
received ten years of general surgical, neurosurgical,
and research training at Columbia/Presbyterian,
New York Hospital, and Oxford. He began work as
the first chief of neurosurgery at Memorial/Sloan
Kettering in New York, then moved to Hershey to
help build Penn State's new medical school. He served
as neurosurgical chief at Harvard's Beth Israel
Hospital for the past five years. His research work
since 1965 – in Oxford, Cornell, Penn State, Harvard,
and Melbourne University – has centred on brain
hormones, especially the transport of hormones from
the body to the brain. Honours include the Borden
Award, the Van Waganen Award, the Markle
Scholarship, and the Macy Faculty Fellowship.

Steve –

The brain belongs
to you, and others
who know the things
you know. go for it!!

Dick

The Fabric of Mind

Richard Bergland

Illustrated by Kati Bromley

Penguin Books Australia Ltd,
487 Maroondah Highway, PO Box 257
Ringwood, Victoria, 3134, Australia
Penguin Books Ltd,
Harmondsworth, Middlesex, England
Penguin Books,
40 West 23rd Street, New York, NY 10010, USA
Penguin Books Canada Ltd,
2801 John Street, Markham, Ontario, Canada
Penguin Books (NZ) Ltd,
182–190 Wairau Road, Auckland 10, New Zealand

First published in Australia by Penguin Books Australia, 1985

Copyright © Richard Bergland, 1985
Illustrations Copyright © Kati Bromley, 1985

Typeset in Century Old Style by Dudley E. King, Melbourne

Made and printed in Australia by
The Dominion Press–Hedges & Bell, Victoria

CIP

Bergland, Richard M., 1932– .
The fabric of mind.

Bibliography.
Includes index.
ISBN 0 14 007460 0.

1. Brain. I. Title.

611'.82

To the genes that were passed into me by Viking
explorers and the memes that were passed into me
by surgical explorers

Contents

There is now little doubt that the brain is a gland; it produces hormones, it has hormone receptors, it is bathed in hormones, hormones run up and down the fibres of individual nerves, and every activity that the brain is engaged in involves hormones.

The implications of this are immense, not only for those who think about thinking – philosophers and scientists – but for virtually every intellectual who reveres the mysterious workings of the mind. Most unsettling to established dogma is the realization that regulatory hormones – the new stuff of thought – are found all over the body.

Can thinking go on outside the brain? Much scientific evidence points to that disturbing, previously unthinkable, possibility.

In this newest intellectual revolution, the disciplines of philosophy, medicine, and science have moved back to a position taken 2,000 years ago by the great Greeks: Plato, Aristotle and Galen. All of them accepted the fact that the brain was a secretory gland. The notion that electricity is the stuff of thought is a very recent idea – less than 200 years old.

My professional life as a neurosurgeon began in this electrical era, a period when scientists and doctors were convinced that electricity was the driving force in the brain. Much that I did in my earlier years was rooted in that premise: electrical circuits in the brain were to be broken or electricity was to be pumped into the brain – all in the name of therapy.

The new view that brain hormones fuel the fires of the mind makes the notion that some good would come out of manipulating the brain's electricity seem as irrational as the blood-letting of Galen (begun in AD 160) or the frontal lobotomies of Egas Moniz (first performed in 1936). Neither Galen nor Moniz lived to see a day of regret for the simple-minded surgical procedures that they performed on their fellow men; I have.

My book is a salute to scientists, a public call to action, and a compendium of new knowledge about the treasury of hormones in the brain.

Richard Bergland
Melbourne, 1985

Paradigms: Pitons of Progress

You have two brains: a left and right.

Modern brain scientists now know that your left brain is your verbal and rational brain; it thinks serially and reduces its thoughts to numbers, letters and words. You might refer to your well-taught, well-read, well-spoken left brain as your *savant*, since whatever wisdom you receive from, or communicate to, the world surrounding you, courses through your left brain.

Your right brain is your non-verbal and intuitive brain; it thinks in patterns, or pictures, composed of 'whole things', and does not comprehend reductions, either numbers, letters or words. You might call your right brain your *mystic*, since its wisdom comes from some hidden source, perhaps a cosmic source. Since your mystic doesn't read, doesn't write, and can't do arithmetic, it can't learn much at school (see Fig. 1.1).

I, too, have a savant-like character living in my left brain and a mystic-like character lurking in the shadows of my right brain. Since my mystic can't write and your mystic can't read, you are hoping that my savant writes well, and I am hoping that your savant reads well; both of us are depending on our left brains.

For my part, my savant has a new-found respect for my right-sided mystic. My left brain – and probably yours – was not taught much respect for the right brain. My teachers heralded rational thought and left-brain reductions. The intuitive thoughts coming from the right brain could not be 'true', they said; real 'truth' could be mathematically expressed and stored in a computer. That viewpoint is the predictable endpoint of left-brain logic and underlies the scientific reductionism that has permeated Western thought for many centuries. But in the past decade, as scientists have changed their thinking about the primary mechanisms of the mind, the right brain, which houses the cosmic wisdom of your mystic, has gained immense intellectual respect: many brain scientists believe that new ideas take root there.

My brains – my savant and mystic – are convinced that the left brain and the right brain are glands and that 'hormones', which are special kinds of wet molecules, modulate every aspect of thinking. The word 'hormone' was first used in 1905 and stems from the Greek word meaning 'to arouse'. The term may be foreign to you; if it has been filed in the word-storage banks in your left brain at all, it is most likely listed under 'sex', 'puberty', or 'the pill', certainly not under 'brain'.

Your two brains may not wish to listen to my brains' new notions. Predictably, they think of themselves as electrically driven computers, 'dry' rather than 'wet'. The notion that the brain is driven by electricity, that electricity is the stuff of thought, is accepted by most of the left brains of the world. It is taught in school, written in books and underlies most thoughts about thinking. So my left brain has a tough job if it is going to get the view that 'the brain is a gland' into your head; it must confront the old view that 'the brain is a computer' and all of the other teachers, writers, and thinkers who gave you that view in the first place.

What does this different point of view mean to you? If you are well, knowing about hormones in the brain could make you smarter; you could use your mind more efficiently. If you are ill, knowing about these hormones could make you feel better; powerful healing forces can flow from your brain to your body, or vice versa.

Knowing that the stuff of thought is not an ethereal spirit or a transient spark can give you more control over your brain; it can help you use it better. Molecules, which you eat or drink and are released when you laugh or cry or exercise, spill into your brain all the time. These determine most of the events in your day: pleasure, love, appetite, satisfaction, joy, sleep, pain, memory, sex, digestion, sadness and anxiety.

The realization that the brain is a gland, controlled by the hormones within it, is less than ten years old. In the past decade, scientists of all kinds have acknowledged that the brain is 'wet'. It is suddenly clear that the unravelling of the mysteries of behaviour can come through a better understanding of brain hormones. But more than that: many kinds of illnesses, especially those related to stress, will be more easily treated by understanding the hormonal signals that move back and forth between the body and the brain.

Less than a decade after scientists began to look at the brain as a gland, psychiatrists are concerned not only with warped relationships but also with crooked molecules. Neurologists are searching for 'missing' hormones, believing that certain brain diseases can be treated by hormone replacement as simply as diabetes is treated with the hormone, insulin. Neurosurgeons have begun to measure the peptides, the tiniest hormones, in the ventricles of the brain; noting that gland tissue transplanted into the brains of animals can cure an experimental Parkinson-like disease, surgeons stand ready to do the same thing for patients with Parkinson's disease. Psychologists are looking for memory peptides, not memory circuits.

Not every scientist and doctor will agree with my notion that the brain is a gland, that 'wet' molecules, endocrine hormones, are the stuff of thought. Many still think of the brain as a 'dry' computer, which is driven by brain electricity. These people will be upset by my belief that the commitment that science made to the understanding of brain electricity did not help patient care. Knowing about brain electricity has given scientists knowledge of the shape of the brain, of its inner circuits, but it has provided physicians who care for patients with brain illnesses very few tools for therapy.

From the traditionally quiet laboratories of the scientists who study brain hormones has erupted a volcano of new ideas about brain illnesses. The same anatomists, physiologists, chemists and cell biologists who were pulled or pushed from each other by brain electricity are now seen huddled together in common laboratories,

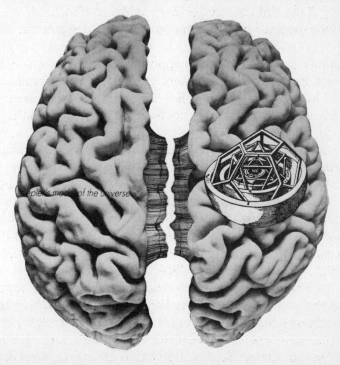

Kepler's model of the universe

Fig. 1.1 The split brain: the left brain thinks verbally; the right brain uses patterns and pictures

projects and multi-disciplinary meetings. These people subscribe to the notion that hormones regulate what the brain eats, when the brain sleeps and how the brain feels. A lack of these hormones may explain brain 'failure', such as the memory loss of senility or the spiritual loss of depression.

Feeding the brain too many such hormones may underlie behavioural addictions, such as those to alcohol, nicotine, coffee and narcotics. These scientists accept the possibility that the brain may produce crooked hormones that can cause crooked behaviour, such as schizophrenia.

By nature, brain scientists and physicians are sceptics. Therefore it is astonishing to note that they herald a new champion: Norman Cousins, a writer who preaches that 'hormones of happiness' may be released by pleasure, joy, humour, and satisfaction. The rejuvenating power of belly laughter, which Cousins found, he first described in America's top medical journal, *The New England Journal of Medicine* and later in a book, *The Anatomy of an Illness*. His journal article received more positive letters than any other article in the journal's history, yet a decade ago his story would have been regarded as that of a mindless quack. Now it is looked upon as the record of a careful observer.

Many of the brain hormones that are important to diseases have long Latin names, forcing doctors to use shorter abbreviations. In years to come, these abbreviations may become part of everyday speech as you hear your friends say:

'I think Phyllis is too fat for diet therapy alone; she needs some CCK.' This abbreviation CCK is shorthand for cholecystokinen, a hormone that limits appetite. Your friends, like the scientists, will avoid the tongue-twister.

Or: 'John is not simply sad, he has a depression that could be easily fixed by CRF.' This abbreviation CRF is used by brain scientists in place of corticotropin releasing factor. In laboratory animals, synthetic CRF can be employed to release the 'hormones of happiness' which may have healed Norman Cousins and could be employed to treat depression.

Or this: 'My Aunt Nellie can't remember a thing; I bet she has exhausted her brain's supply of AVP.' Arginine vasopressin, called AVP, is a brain hormone that improves memory and sharpens learning in many laboratory situations. Many predict that AVP will be employed in future years to treat patients with senile dementia.

Before these hope-filled conversations become everyday realities, many revolutionary changes must occur in the way patients and doctors view the stuff of thought. Yet without much doubt, those changes have begun.

Few non-scientists comprehend the significance of the simple statement 'the brain is a gland', but time may bear out my prediction that this phrase will be of more benefit to mankind than the more succinct statement $E=MC^2$. That cold calculation separated person from person and unchained as much violence in people's hearts as it did in the heart of the atom. In the centuries that follow, people will be involved in establishing links between the hormones of the brain and human behaviour. The scope of this undertaking is immense, and entirely positive.

Both those still committed to the scientific reductionism of the West and those devoted to the holistic view more acceptable to the East will gain by understanding that hormones, not electrical sparks, are the prime moving forces of the brain. Those in the West directed towards more precise correlations between newly discovered brain hormones and old, poorly understood diseases can be more sharply focused; they can quickly apply on-the-shelf techniques of endocrinology to their reductionism. Those in the East can go forward knowing that the new knowledge concerning the ebb and flow of hormones between the brain and the body supports much of what they have taught for centuries. Religion – meditation and prayer – is suddenly in the mainstream of scientific concern.

Learning about the history of brain science and about some of its current problems may change the way you think not only about your brain, but also about the institutions in our society that are dedicated to the care and feeding of our brains.

Hospitals, the places that care for the brains of those who are ill, must surely change as a result of the new knowledge about the brain. Both those who are ill and the doctors who care for them have been disserviced by the scientists who for more than a century have been preaching the importance of the paradigm that the brain is an electrically driven computer. The new information about brain hormones should bring help and hope to those shackled by brain illnesses, those who have taken their brains or those of their loved ones to hospitals to find neither cure nor explanation.

Perhaps what is more important, universities, the places which feed the brains of those who are well, will also address the issues that spring from the new knowledge about the mechanisms of the mind. I hope my comments will lend support to the millions of students who take their query-filled brains to academic institutions, often to be turned off or driven away.

In the effort to understand the human mind there has been continuous tension between the institutions that gain comfort from the security of the centre and the individuals who seek the uncertain, productive excitement of the edge. To look in at one's own brain in a new way while looking out at the academic institutions that at once feed and suck from the human brain should benefit scholars of all kinds. 'The known is finite, the unknown infinite; intellectually we stand on an island in the midst of an illimitable ocean of inexplicability. Our business in every generation is to reclaim a little more land,' wrote T. H. Huxley in 1887.

No matter what you do in your life, you stand with me on such an island. We both recognize the treasury of the interrelated answers at the centre and the magnetism of the unanswered questions visible from the shoreline. As our island of knowledge grows, our shoreline of wonder should expand. But the treasury of information at the centre must be defended by our mates – our institutions. And the shorelines of wonder must be explored by individuals – by you and me.

A special kind of tension at once links us to and separates us from our intellectual institutions. It may grow from this: you and I are meant to find new 'truths' at the shoreline; the institutions are supposed to keep 'truths' at the centre.

Even greater tension will develop between those who stand at the centre defending the old paradigm that the brain is an electrically driven computer and those who find themselves on a new shoreline advocating the new view that the brain is a hormonally modulated gland. It is this competition that instigates the 'Shoreline of Wonder' sections which end each chapter; I hope these written parentheses will encourage those readers who reach the new shoreline to look at social, philosophical and religious horizons in a new way.

Shoreline of Wonder

As we think, something must float like a shuttlecock from the right side of the brain to the left, and vice versa. We could call this stuff electricity or information or ideas or models for thought. In India it might be called 'citta'. But none of these terms is perfectly suited for the complex interrelated thoughts about the brain that we will be considering. 'Idea-chord' might be a good choice; it comes from Douglas Hofstadter's statement in *Godel, Escher and Bach*:

Perhaps what differentiates highly creative thoughts from ordinary ones is some combined sense of beauty, simplicity, and harmony – deeply related ideas are often superficially disparate. The analogy to chords is natural: physically close notes are harmonically distant and harmonically close notes are physically distant . . . harmonious *idea-chords* [my italics] are often widely separated as measured on an imaginary keyboard of concepts.

'Memes', a neologism invented by Richard Dawkins in his book *The Selfish Gene*, would be a trendy descriptive term for these shuttling thoughts. Dawkins emphasized the importance of genes to cells, but argued that memes exercise the same kind of control in the mind. Even though they are powerful, genes have not been the shaping force of our culture. The genetic distinction of Beethoven or Einstein is lost in three or four generations; their splendid genes, once poured into the extraordinarily large vat of the human genetic pool, are lost forever. But the memes of Beethoven and Einstein, their good ideas, are passed from one generation to another and have an eternal significance. All animals are gene dependent. But the evolution of our culture, of our civilization, is meme dependent.

Genes are body shapers, actually cell shapers, which may infect the cell; once inside, they cause it to 'selfishly' replicate more and more identical genes. Memes, Dawkins contends, are mind shapers, which pass from brain to brain like an infectious virus. Not all of the ideas that pass from one brain to another brain, however, are good ideas; some are mistakes. These I call 'mismemes'.

'Paradigm' is another possibility and certainly the best term for the models for thought about the brain. Thomas Kuhn describes the term in his book *The Structure of Scientific Revolutions*:

Without commitment to a paradigm there can be no science . . . the study of paradigms is what prepares a student for membership in a particular scientific community. Men whose research is based on shared paradigms are committed to the same rules and standards for scientific practice . . . scientific revolutions are inaugurated by a growing sense that an existing paradigm has ceased to function adequately in the exploration of an aspect of nature.

I believe the existing paradigm about the brain has ceased to function adequately.

2

The Power of the Paradigm

*I*t is easy to trace the path that Sir Edmund Hillary took up Mount Everest; the base camps that he set up have become shrines to those who followed him. Many of the pitons, the small metal spikes driven into the mountain walls by climbers, can still be found, defining the path along which his rope-linked climbers ascended.

It is also easy to trace the path that scholars have taken in their effort to understand the brain. The paradigms that scientists have put forward on the mechanics of the mind stand as pitons of intellectual progress; each new paradigm has lifted our understanding of the mind to a higher plateau, and these models for thought chart a course of mankind's most challenging intellectual ascent.

My book will lead you along the ascending paths that the study of the mind has taken. Along each path intellectual base camps have been constructed by teams of climbers who decided it was a propitious time to break camp and move to a higher place. Few if any of these new base camps were found by teams of scouts; most of the upward steps were taken first by people acting alone.

Kuhn describes such steps well in his book about scientific revolutions, pointing out again and again that the plans of future scientific development determined by the group seldom lead to paradigm shifts. The dents in the frontiers of science, the new paradigms, have almost always been made by lone scouts.

A paradigm shift, a movement to a higher intellectual plateau, occurs when a lone scout returns with information about a new path. The scout must convince those in the base camp that it is time to move up.

The debate will be carried on by the group, always linked by a common concern for receiving information, connecting it, deciding if it is 'true', and then answering all possible criticisms. These intellectual functions depend upon verbal communications, and modern brain scientists affirm that such work is performed by the left brain. Letters, words and numbers are stored there and, indeed, all 'group mentality' could be regarded as a linkage of left brains.

By contrast, the lonely Viking-like risk-takers who discovered the better paths for intellectual ascent were generally driven by the pattern-dependent mental qualities of searching, probing, balancing and questioning. It was Roger Sperry who first affirmed that pattern-dependent thinking takes place in the right brain, and for this discovery he was given the Nobel Prize in 1981.

If mind mechanisms in the right brain guide the scouts who implant the pitons of progress during intellectual ascents, it would be expected that they would act alone, since right brains, unable to communicate with one another, cannot link themselves together.

The importance of paradigms was discovered first by Pythagoras. The first scientific paradigm, and the second, were generated in his mind.

Pythagoras was born 582 years before Christ on the tiny Greek Island of Samos. He received scant education, but nonetheless at the time of his death, at the age of eighty-two, he had laid the cornerstones for both art and science.

Pythagoras was the first to understand the scientific principles of harmonious music. His tools of inquiry were simple: the stretched strings of the lute, the favourite musical instrument of the day. He established that a string vibrating along its full length produces a constant note. Another vibrating string, stretched to the same tension, which is one-half as long, or one-third as long, or one-fourth as long, produces a harmonious sound. Any other length of vibrating string produces discordant sound.

These simple experiments wrestled from nature a simple secret that had eluded musicians for centuries. It was the first scientific paradigm. Music, until Pythagoras, had come from plucked single strings. His discovery of these mathematical principles allowed two musical notes, or a thousand musical notes, to be played together in harmony.

From that time forward, music had a language. It could be read by the eye, not only heard by the ear. It could be composed, copied, learned and passed from generation to generation. His scientific discovery established the only truly universal language, a breathtaking achievement, yet so simple.

Pythagoras constructed another paradigm that altered mathematics forever after. Again he brought order to disorder by simple, pattern-dependent observations.

Sensing the utility of the right-angled set square that had been used by builders in construction projects for many centuries, he discovered constant numerical relationships between its three sides. No matter what shape or size, if the length of the longest arm of the triangle, the hypotenuse, was squared (length times length), it would equal the sum of the squared lengths of the other two sides of the triangle.

This helped builders immensely; they would waste less wood. Knowing that the length of a vertical beam was 6 feet and the length of its right-angled horizontal joining member was 8 feet, for example, the builder could saw a joining timber that was precisely 10 feet long. The calculation was simple: $6 \times 6 = 36$. Then $8 \times 8 = 64$. Adding 36 to 64 gave 100. The square root of 100 is 10.

Why was this simple observation so important? Not because it allowed bigger, taller buildings and more efficient carpentry. The Pythagorean theorem proved that there is an internal consistency between numbers. It gave the numbers of equations, for example, $6 \times 6 = 36$, a reality of their own. In a stroke, theoretical relationships were given a substance as solid as bricks or wood.

After Pythagoras, theoretical thought was possible for the first time. The mind could now fly into the world of the intangible; it could conceptualize for the first time, invent paradigms, knowing that such models possessed a substance of their own. Again, a breathtaking achievement.

A disciple of Pythagoras's named Empedocles (500–430 BC) and his students saw that everything Pythagoras had accomplished involved numbers. They constructed a religion based on the premise that numbers were the building blocks of the universe: by their mystical, eternal relationships numbers controlled all humans, gods and demons. Avid geometrists, they concluded that the circle was the perfect two-dimensional form and the sphere the perfect three-dimensional form. The circle and the sphere were symmetrical in every way: each half was the same no matter how they were sliced, and every point on a circle or a sphere was the same as every other point. To them this was perfection.

They saw that right-angled triangles could be brought together to form an equilateral triangle that would fit exactly both within and around a circle. The simple juxtaposition illustrated in Fig. 2.1 linked the eternal truth of the Pythagorean theorem to the perfect circle, enhancing the importance of both.

These scholars concluded that right-angled triangles were the basic building blocks of nature; they could be brought together to form different two-dimensional shapes, which in turn could be brought together to form three-dimensional atoms. Four such atoms shared in the perfection of the sphere – they would fit both within and around it – leading them to conclude that these perfect atoms comprised all things on earth.

Watching a log burn, Empedocles and his followers could see that it was a combination of four different substances. First, fire came out of it. Second, smoke, a kind of air, came from it. Third, in wet logs water came from the end of the log as it burned. Fourth, when all of these things had gone away, earth, the ashes, remained. Since they had ascertained that the tiny atoms with the triangular shapes could only form four objects, they jumped to the conclusion that the four elements so obviously joined together in the log by nature were the four natural elements.

Fire, said Empedocles, was composed of the pyramid-like atom, the four-sided tetrahedron. Earth was composed of six-sided cubes. Air was composed of eight-sided octahedrons. Water was composed of twenty-sided icosohedrons.

The group not only linked one of their triangular-skinned atoms to each of earth's four elements, but also assigned forces of love and strife to them. The good forces of love could bring fire and

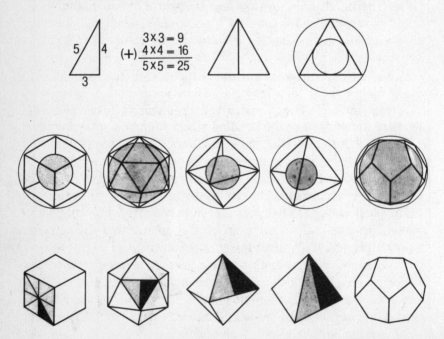

Fig. 2.1 The circle, the sphere and four of the Platonic bodies shared the eternal relationships of the right-angled triangle; the dodecahedron did not

water together to form steam; the bad forces of strife would make it impossible for fire and water to co-exist; fires could be snuffed out by dashing them with water. The good forces would bring earth and water together to form clay, then pots. The opposing force would separate earth and water into dry land and the ocean. The seasons of the macrocosm and the humours of the microcosm were both determined by the coming together of these atomic forces. The four-square relationship between the four elements described in Fig. 2.2 has been hung on classroom walls for many more centuries than the periodic tables of the atomic elements that you memorized in school.

It was a rational assessment of how things might be, the kind of paradigm that could easily be passed from left brain to left brain, especially if each person in the group was dedicated to the notion that numbers ruled the world. This made the leap into the world of self-deception much easier. Once this mismeme was implanted in mathematically fertilized left brains, it would flourish, as indeed it did. It survived in the left brains of those who followed Empedocles for nearly 2,000 years.

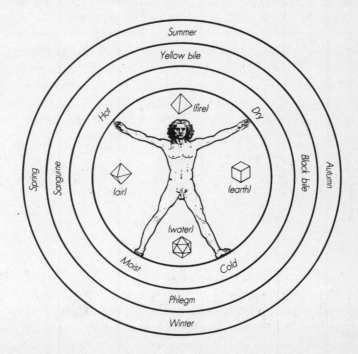

Fig. 2.2 The ancient Greeks thought the forces of 'love' brought Platonic bodies together to form the four humours and the four seasons

One 'truth' that was discovered by the Pythagoreans was not taught to those outside their school. It was hidden as a secret because it did not fit their triangle-based paradigm. The mathematicians there found an atom, the dodecahedron, which was formed not by triangular planes, but by twelve pentagons. It was more like a sphere than any of their other atoms. It could also fit perfectly into and around a sphere.

But the dodecahedron did not contain any right-angled triangles and could not share in the mystical qualities of that form. One of the instructors, Hippasus, revealed this secret to outsiders but later died in a shipwreck. Justice, said Empedocles, more concerned about the security of the secret than the security of the fellow.

The Pythagoreans whom Empedocles led conjured up another false notion that there were four humours in man that were linked to the four natural substances. These were black bile, yellow bile, phlegm and sanguine. Each of these was formed by the forces of love or strife interacting with fire, air, earth or water.

The belief in Empedocles's four humours passed into the minds of great physicians such as Hippocrates and Galen and led them off the track. Both of these men came to espouse the four humours and this mistaken belief, an outgrowth of the Pythagorean mismeme, permeated medicine in the dark ages.

But medicine was not the only intellectual discipline that was misdirected by a belief that Platonic bodies were nature's building blocks. Philosophy, religion, indeed, astronomy were held in chains by this mismeme. It was taught in all the schools in the Western world from the time of Empedocles until the Renaissance, a long-lasting demonstration of the power of the paradigm.

Shoreline of Wonder

Adam and Eve, placed in the centre of man's first physical garden, failed to honour their Creator; theirs was the first religious 'sin'. Empedocles, placed in the centre of man's first intellectual garden, failed to honour creative thought; his was the first scientific 'sin'.

Modern brain scientists acknowledge that the functions of the human brain are 'split': some tasks are performed in the right hemisphere and others in the left. Pattern recognition is performed by the right brain and verbal tasks, such as reading, writing, speaking and hearing, by the left brain. Modern-day dynamic brain scans are able to confirm Sperry's 'split-brain' observations with remarkable precision; during reading, for example, only a small part of the left brain is at work.

Since the two paradigms of Pythagoras were so clearly dependent upon patterns – the pattern of movement of musical strings and the pattern of lines and angles in triangles – it can be assumed with confidence that his right brain was at work during the invention of his paradigms. But his right brain, like all right brains, could not communicate. It could neither hear, speak, read nor write.

It is no accident that mankind's first paradigms involved patterns; it is difficult to conceive of models for thought that do not involve patterns in one way or another.

Two modern paradigms emphasize the importance of patterns. August Kekule (1829–96), after dreaming of a snake that had swallowed its tail, conceived of a circle of carbon atoms coming together in the form of a benzene ring. This simple pattern is the basis for all organic chemistry, indeed, the basis for all organic life in plants and animals. James Watson and Francis Crick actually cut out patterned pieces of cardboard to discover that the genetic code of all living cells was formed by a twisted double helix of DNA.

The right brain, the body's only pattern maker, must have been involved in all of this. If you look back two millennia to Pythagoras, one century to Kekule, or three decades to Watson and Crick, you see the same thing: patterns influencing the direction of new thoughts. In every age and for every new paradigm, the right brain's contribution is crucial. Once new models for thought are constructed by the brain, they are held up against the reality of the outside world and the question asked, 'Does the model fit?' In this model-verification process, again the right brain must be most responsible, especially if a pattern of some kind is involved.

Thus the non-communicating right brain serves dually as the creator of pattern-dependent paradigms and the verifier of paradigm reliability.

In group mentality some exclusion of the right brain must occur; this side of the brain does not involve itself in verbal discussions. A new paradigm arising in the right brain of a person is regarded as a 'dream' by the group; only a model that can be described in words and numbers can pass as a meme between the interconnected left brains of the group.

This phenomenon, and its disastrous consequences, is especially obvious among those who followed Pythagoras: they formed the first committee and were bound together by their left brains as any committee must be. Guided by left-brain thinking, they were concerned more with well-spoken answers and well-calculated numbers. New unexpressable and uncalculable paradigms were regarded as untrue dreams, the model-verification process of the right brain was excluded from the group mentality and with that exclusion, honest questions about group-honoured answers became impossible. Soon the group gave answers from their group-connected left brains before there were questions or new models from any individual right brains. They piled one unquestioned answer on top of another. With no right brains to construct new models on those of Pythagoras and no right brains encouraged to ask, 'Does the model fit?' the committee could neither build new paradigms nor verify old ones.

After Empedocles, many centuries passed before the questioning spirit of the right mind was again allowed to participate in scientific inquiry. Science became a cataloguing endeavour, geared neatly to the abilities of the left brain. Both Plato and Aristotle accepted the 'burning log' breakdown of the natural elements, and Aristotle gave the atom with pentagonal skin, the dodecahedron, a God-like significance.

Plato and Aristotle were bright men, by the measure of most scholars, the most intelligent teacher/student team ever to walk on earth. Yet both of them were caught up by the humbug of the Pythagorean atomists.

In the history of brain science, the institutions that have been responsible for keeping the 'truth' have set in place bureaucracies that have been similar to that established by Empedocles. But the individuals who find the 'truth' have different attributes from the institutions that keep it.

The finders can trace their intellectual heritage to Pythagoras who was concerned with questions, the unknown, the future and the next paradigm.

The keepers can trace their lineage to the school of Empedocles and the security-minded bureaucrats concerned with answers, the known, the past, the last paradigm.

Finders are leaders; it is the right brain that leads leaders to the edge. It is the left brain that keeps keepers at the centre.

3

Questions, not Answers

What Socrates (470–399 BC) thought about the brain we will never know. He was not a writer. Most of what we know about his thoughts comes to us through the writing of Plato, his student. But in discussing paradigms, and the development of new paradigms, we must acknowledge that it was Socrates who first said that questions are more important than answers. Only questions, he said, could keep people intellectually honest.

It was his ability to frame questions that kindled the intellectual revolution that began in Athens 2,400 years ago. His questions were concerned entirely with social, ethical and political relationships between people. He thought that the study of nature was below the dignity of a philosopher. One of his students wrote that Socrates considered the astronomy that captivated the minds of other Greeks of that era a waste of time.

What was the fate of Socrates, the first great question-asker? His wife regarded him as a lazy, unemployed, and unreliable ne'er-do-well. He published nothing despite his prodigious mental activities. His concerns for a better society went unheeded as his own city crumbled into chaos. This man, acknowledged as our intellectual father, was judged by his peers to be a menace to the youth of Athens and asked to go away and kill himself.

What went wrong between Socrates and his institutional colleagues we can never know for certain, but from Plato's description in the *Apology*, the Athenian city fathers wanted answers, not questions. Transferring answers from one brain to another has fairly predictable consequences: answers are safe. Infecting young minds with questions is hazardous; it is impossible to predict the outcome, and some of those infected may decide that they prefer the questions to the answers. Society, in Athens or anywhere, is most predictable and hence most controllable if it is strung together by answers.

Why didn't Socrates write? The world did not receive one word from his pen. It is certainly obvious that questions reigned in his mind. If you recall his statement, 'I know nothing' and his repeated question, 'What do you mean?', you must wonder with me if he wasn't blessed with a weakened left cerebral hemisphere. The written information that comes to such people cannot be well received. They are regarded by modern schoolteachers as 'dyslexics'.

Socrates may have been the first of many great question-askers who were right-brain dominant. The most well known is Leonardo da Vinci (AD 1452–1519) whose mirror-writing is proof of dyslexia. Leonardo's problem became his creative advantage. His private diaries record clearly that questions dominated his brain, but they were not seen until a century after his death. His diaries contained pictures that were often drawn one on top of the other, each a clear description of an important question about the world, but few linked in orderly fashion. The words that were appended to his pictures were all written backwards.

Leonardo's mirror-writing is shown in Fig. 3.1 in his drawing of the ventricles, the hollow, fluid-filled space that is in the centre of the brain. Leonardo discerned this pattern by filling the ventricles with melted wax; once he had removed the brain tissue, the form of the ventricles was maintained. The process that he employed is very similar to the casting technique sculptors employ to form bronze statues.

A second giant of biology whose mind's eye was doomed to reside in the right brain was John Hunter (AD 1728–93), my greatest hero and modern medicine's most prolific original thinker. Hunter never entered the portals of a school as a child, even

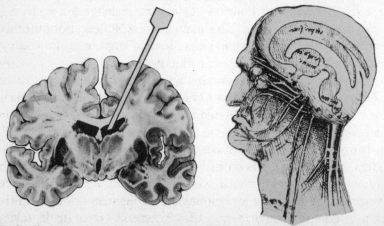

Fig. 3.1 The first drawing of the ventricles, the fluid-filled spaces in the centre of the brain. To show their shape, Leonardo put a needle in the ventricles, filled them with wax and removed the brain

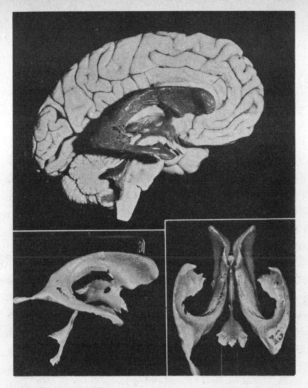

Fig. 3.2 Casts of the human ventricles

though schooling was a strong tradition in his well-educated upper-class Scottish family. Sent by his family to work as the scut boy in his elder brother's London laboratory, Hunter did what any dyslexic must do: observe for himself. Single-handedly, he began the revolution in biological thought that is still going on. He is now regarded as the father of surgery, infectious diseases, endocrinology and experimental biology. Yet, like Socrates, Hunter did not leave a written intellectual legacy, and it is believed that some of the things that were 'written' by him were actually ghost-written by his close associates in an effort to polish his academic reputation.

John Hunter secured most of his new thoughts in thousands of glass bottles that he filled with his delicate dissections of the patterns nature used to form the body. This collection was partially destroyed in the bombing of London, but much of it remains as the central portion of the Hunterian Museum in London. The museum contains many casts of human ventricles, which were produced by using the same casting techniques that Leonardo had used in the brain to discern the pattern of blood vessels. These eye-catching statutes are shown in Fig. 3.2.

The best universities in the world still employ the Socratic method of teaching, still insist, as Socrates did, that real learning will only occur if questions precede answers. The best teachers still recognize that it is the probing, questioning mind that allows one to survive independently in the world. The best researchers in the world recognize the weakness of the left hemisphere; they still worry about getting the right answer to the wrong question.

Are the smartest among us those with the best 'patterns' in their right brains? Can they hold up better patterns against the same outer world that you and I see to generate better questions, decisions and new thoughts? Was the ability to form better patterns the secret to the intellectual success of Socrates, Leonardo and Hunter?

Another of my heroes, Charles Sherrington (AD 1857–1952), is regarded as the father of experimental neurology. He once remarked to Howard Florey, who discovered penicillin, 'Research is essentially a conversation with nature and like any good conversation, good research hinges on good questions.'

Socrates taught Sherrington that; Socrates taught us all that the answer can be good only if the question is good.

Shoreline of Wonder

A few times in this book I have used the word 'truth', most often taking care to put it in quotation marks. As Thomas Kuhn points out in his book on scientific revolutions, 'truth' is funny stuff. Not one, but many of the paradigms that have been judged to be 'true' in the past contained 'false' observations. It is now established that Mendel, the father of genetics, calculated on mathematical tables the changes that would occur in fruit flies before he did the experiments. Though a religious priest, he fudged his data to fit more neatly with the paradigm that he knew to be 'true'. Some of the skulls that anthropologists have 'found' and described as evolutionary links are outright frauds, and again these were presented to buttress a paradigm that was for the greatest part 'true'. Kuhn and other historians are remarkably charitable about such deceptions, acknowledging that the fervour of Western scientists to establish a new 'truth' commonly leads them to these embarrassments. They take a kind philosophical view that the human mind can never actually 'contain the truth'; it can only describe a paradigm, a best estimate. The best estimates must be incomplete and, in that sense, are not wholly true. But just as frequent are omissions of troublesome 'truths', which if accepted would make belief in the greater paradigm impossible.

Lamentably, I have lived in academic institutions now noted for scientific fraud, and in recent years have wrestled personally with the issues of 'truth' in my own science. Since my conclusions about the matter entail a respect for questions, rather than answers, it is appropriate to include these observations here.

I have been interested in the pituitary gland, the tiny bean-shaped organ that hangs from the brain into a special cup in the base of the skull, for the past twenty years (see Fig. 3.3).

I am not certain what force, or meme, came into my life that led me to go deeper into the relationships between the brain and the pituitary, but eventually I came to the point where I knew as much about this minuscule part of the body as anybody on earth. I say that without conceit, and would tell any young person that with enough dedication, focus, gumption and time anybody can reach and shape a frontier.

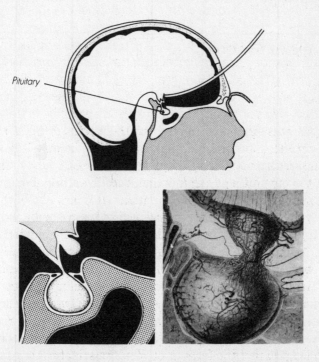

Pituitary

Fig. 3.3 The pituitary gland resides in a bony cup, yet hangs from the base of the brain by a stalk, much like an apple from its stem

In writing down my observations for the journal, *Science*, it dawned on me that the 'truth' concerning brain-pituitary relationships could not be moved easily from my left brain, where I had stored my observations, to the pages that I was writing. If the 'truth' about this topic existed anywhere, it was in my brain. But then I realized that the organized thoughts, the paradigms, that were in my brain were sometimes all answers and at other times all questions. The paradigms seemed to bounce back and forth between their question-phase and their answer-phase. Although I felt compelled to push the paradigms out of my left brain through my right hand, I knew that only the paradigms that were formed of answers would make sense to the editors, reviewers and readers. I experienced an epistemological crisis, knowing that my written words were not constantly 'true', even though they embodied my best attempt to push the 'truth' out.

Most unsettling was the personal realization that there was no steady 'truth'. Every answer would produce more questions which would produce more answers. In the answer-phase, concepts could be more easily described, but even then an answer that seemed correct in the morning could seem incorrect in the evening in the light of some fact I had forgotten to include in the morning thinking. When the 'truth' was more in the question-phase, there was much more intellectual progress. Answers needed links, one with another. That required almost a mathematically precise understanding of both the anatomy and the chemistry of the issue in focus. Any answer that didn't fit was quickly dismissed. Questions, by contrast, did not have to interlock. They could be juxtaposed in odd ways. By position alone they could induce the accidental cross-linkages that make intellectual evolution – creative thought – possible. Questions were not quickly dismissed; they could hang around for days on end, totally unrelated to other thoughts, but influencing them nonetheless.

It was about then that I realized the creative advantage of Leonardo: if progress was my goal, I must keep the questions in my brain as much as possible. That method of thinking would afford me a much better chance of untangling the puzzle that was before me. And at that time I realized why Leonardo 'thought' in pictures, and why John Hunter collected his thoughts in bottles; both were convenient ways to store questions.

Most of my questions about the pituitary have been stored in a single photograph (Fig. 3.4). This is a modern scanning electron-micrograph of the pituitary of a rhesus monkey. All the blood vessels are filled with plastic, but the pituitary tissue and the

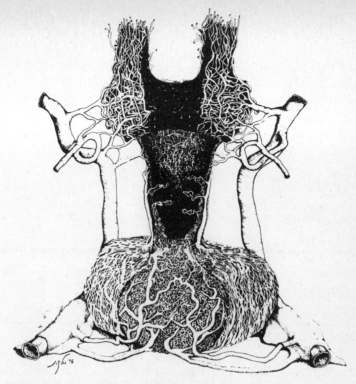

Fig. 3.4 A cast of the blood vessels of a monkey's pituitary, showing that there are many pathways for blood into but not out of the pituitary

surrounding bone have been digested with a lye-like solution. It is a cast, a modern-day version of the technique employed by Leonardo and Hunter.

This picture has been reproduced in many textbooks, yet it confounds me; indeed, it confounds most of the scientists who know most about the pituitary. It shows that the pituitary is extremely vascular; there are many pathways by which blood can get into the pituitary, but very few pathways that can carry blood to the surrounding veins. It suggests that the pituitary should explode; blood can get in but not out.

Not months but years of my life have been spent pondering the pituitary blood vessels which form this elegant cast. I can see the anatomical pattern, but I can't discern the physiological pattern.

Out of respect for the pattern-dependent questions of Socrates, Leonardo and Hunter and for my own unanswered questions about the pituitary has come the conviction that if the brain is to look at itself and know itself, the questioning mirror should be held by the left hand of the pattern-forming right brain.

Academies: Places with Answers

No contrast in academic history is as vivid as the fates of Socrates and his student Plato (427-347 BC). Socrates's awful death came in large measure from his incessant questions. Plato's glorious success came from his skilled answers. The same city fathers who reviled Socrates came to revere Plato.

After Socrates drank the hemlock, Plato left Athens (in 399 BC) and travelled to many places in the Mediterranean, probably Egypt, but more certainly Italy and Sicily. In Sicily he studied in the school of the Pythagoreans, and when he returned to Athens in 387 BC he set up his own school in a garden called the Academy. He was so taken by the Pythagorean concept that atoms with triangular skins were the building blocks of nature that these mythical molecules became central to much of his teaching. For many centuries after, they were known as 'Platonic bodies' even though the concept did not originate with Plato.

The garden school that Plato established in Athens began in 380 BC and continued to teach students without a break until AD 529, a span of 909 years. It was in this garden that Aristotle spent twenty years at the feet of Plato.

Plato had all the skills that one would expect to come from the left brain; he was an orderly thinker, a gifted writer, a splendid organizer and a masterful politician. He was not a scientist, yet he was the first to pronounce to the world that he knew what the brain did. His conclusion was strange, almost ludicrous, but like many of the mismemes that came from the Pythagoreans, it persisted for nearly 2,000 years and had immense social consequences.

Plato was an avid astronomer, very different from Socrates, his teacher. He became familiar with the movement of the heavenly bodies and pronounced that the heavens were clearly alive: they moved. Moreover, they moved perfectly, in circles. As he believed that the universe itself was perfect, it must be of perfect shape; the only perfect shape he had learned from his Pythagorean education was the sphere. He leapt to the conclusion that stars moved in perfect circles in a perfectly spherical universe.

The circular movement that Plato gave to the stars took on a scientific, philosophical and religious significance that held thoughtful people in intellectual chains for 1,900 years.

The church accepted Plato's view that only the heavenly bodies could move in never-ending circles. When Michael Servetus pronounced in AD 1553 that blood could also move by 'circulation', he was burned at the stake.

Copernicus, born in AD 1470, knew for certain in his fortieth year that the sun, not the earth, was the centre of our universe. Knowing that the church adamantly held to Plato's view, Copernicus was slow to publicly describe his discovery. His book was published thirty years later, in the year of his death: AD 1543.

Galileo, nearly a century later, supported Copernicus but was forced in AD 1633 to write:

I must altogether abandon the false opinion that the sun is the centre of the world and immovable, and that the earth is not the centre of the world, and moves, and I must not hold, defend, or teach in any way whatsoever, verbally or in writing, the said doctrine, after it had been notified to me that the said doctrine was contrary to Holy Scripture.

No other mismeme has had the impact of Plato's false notion that the universe was a perfect sphere and that stars moved in perfect circles.

It was Plato's belief in the perfect sphere that led him to conclude that the rational soul of man, 'the divinest part of us', must be in the brain. Why? Quite simply, because the head was spherical in shape. Having placed 'the divinest part' of man in the sphere of the head, Plato assumed that genetic material must be formed in that place, and he postulated that the brain was the organ that produced semen.

The view that the male brain produced semen was a mismeme that passed from brain to brain for centuries. The proof of this paradigm's longevity is given in the Leonardo cartoon drawn 1,900 years later (see Fig. 4.1). That anatomical drawing defines an open, continuous pathway that could carry sperm from the brain, through the spinal cord and a fictitious tube into the penis of a copulating male and into the female vagina.

This paradigm gave the female brain no role at all and regarded women only as flower pots for male seeds. The acceptance of this paradigm led to the exclusion of women from the governance of academic, religious and governmental institutions for 2,000 years or longer. This is perhaps the best evidence that the form of our culture and our civilization can be shaped – or misshaped – by the scientific views concerning the brain.

Plato was the first to assign a function to the human brain and suggested that it was a secretory organ, indeed, a gland. He was correct, but for the wrong reasons.

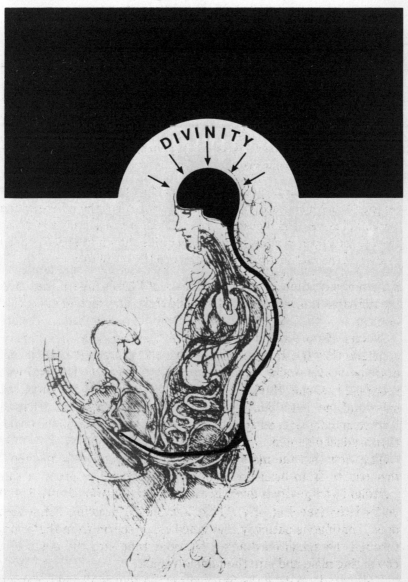

Fig. 4.1 Leonardo's anatomical drawings show an open continuous pathway from the spinal cord to the penis, reflecting the view that semen was formed in the brain and carried down the spinal cord

On a tiny island called Cos, 500 miles to the East of Athens, lived another Greek who would profoundly influence medical thought. This man, Hippocrates (460–370 BC), was not given to writing, much like Socrates. Most of his thoughts were passed along by the students who gathered at his side. From those students comes the following statement about the brain:

Men ought to know that from the brain, and from the brain only, arise our pleasures, joys, laughter and jests, as well as our sorrows, pains, griefs, and tears. Through it . . . we . . . think, see, hear, and distinguish the ugly from the beautiful, the bad from the good, the pleasant from the unpleasant.

Inexplicably, the very correct view of the brain held by those in Cos never made it to the school that Plato established in Athens.

Plato's view was that of 'hard' science; it gave the brain something physical to do: produce semen. Hippocrates's paradigm was that of a 'soft' scientist; he involved it with joy and sorrow, ugliness and beauty, goodness and badness, and pleasantness and unpleasantness. Since then, a 'hard'/'soft', scientific/spiritual dichotomy has persisted between Western and Eastern brain scientists. Only now, in the past decade, has a scientific reconciliation begun between these polarized viewpoints.

How could Plato, who was correct about so many things, be so wrong about the brain? Like the committees of Empedocles, those who surrounded Plato made no experimental effort to verify his well-described paradigms. The right brain was excluded; the left brain's well-worded, well-calculated descriptions were 'true', and the greatest writers were enthroned as the greatest thinkers. Plato's writing skills guaranteed that his unquestioned answer about the brain would persist as a mismeme.

But criticisms of Plato's views about the brain should be generously couched. The modern view that the brain's *raison d'être* is to produce electricity now seems to be as erroneous as Plato's view that the brain was created to produce semen. Both are examples of scientific observations described so well in written words and numbers – in reductions – that question-asking right brains concerned with holistic patterns have no say.

Aristotle (384–322 BC) was born into a wealthy family in Macedonia, an area in northern Greece. His father, the king's physician, sent Aristotle to the Academy in Athens, and he studied there, with Plato, for the next twenty years.

When Plato died in 348 BC, Aristotle left Athens, moved to the coast of what is now Turkey, and lived on a tiny island, Lesbos. Four years later he was asked by his father's employer, King Phillip, to return to Macedonia to teach the king's son, Alexander, later known as Alexander the Great.

After his pupil set off on his conquests, Aristotle returned to Athens and established a school, the Lyceum, several miles from Plato's Academy. He became the father of biology and even today his scientific accomplishments are heralded, yet he gave his students, both in science and philosophy, an erroneous notion about the stuff of thought that created immense and long-lasting confusion. One of the graduates of the Lyceum was selected to head the libraries in Alexandria and carried Aristotle's mismeme there. These wrong ideas were defended as the 'truth' by the librarians there for nearly 600 years and became the cornerstone for both science and religion. In recounting the development and the preservation of Aristotle's mistake there are many lessons for modern brain biologists.

Aristotle was a keen and careful observer who insisted that he join in the grisly task of animal dissection. His independent searching in all fields of nature, especially biology, has not been matched. Alexander the Great gave him 1,000 servants for his biological laboratory, and with this help he dissected more than 540 different species. From these studies he produced textbooks of embryology, anatomy and reproduction that remained without equal for 1,900 years. In them, he described a 'hierarchy of creatures' that was very close to the principles of evolution enunciated by Charles Darwin in 1856.

Aristotle differs from his predecessors immensely: none of them valued the orderly accumulation of anatomical observations. Indeed, Plato had taught his students that the senses could only deceive; to him, pure contemplation, unencumbered by observation of any kind, was the only method by which man could know the 'truth'. By emphasizing the value of biological observation, Aristotle laid the cornerstone of biological science, much as Pythagoras had done for mathematics nearly two centuries before.

Despite his penchant for observation, however, Aristotle accepted without any evidence many theories on the make-up of the universe that had been passed from Pythagoras to Empedocles and to his teacher, Plato.

Like his ancestors, Aristotle was convinced that the heavens were spherical and 'alive'. The life he believed to be in the heavens was the prime moving force for the universe, his famous *primum mobile*.

As Plato had done, he accepted the notion that the earth was composed of four kinds of atoms with triangular skins. Although the atoms of the heavenly bodies remained in perfect order, the earthly elements were generally disordered. Yet earthly bodies had a natural tendency to assume orderly positions based upon their divinity, or nobility. To him, the heavens were more noble than fire, fire more noble than air, air more noble than water, and water more noble than earth. The 'holiness' of heaven began in Plato's mind, but it was a key portion of Aristotle's philosophy. His support of this concept guaranteed that it would be accepted later by the librarians of Alexandria and thereafter by religions of many kinds, for both librarians and priests held Aristotle in the highest esteem. His concept of the *primum mobile* in the heavens closely resembles the Judaeo-Christian concept of a 'God in heaven'; Thomas Aquinas (AD 1225–74) made the fact that there was a prime moving force at the edge of the universe his first proof for the existence of God.

Aristotle's myth-filled view of earth and heaven set the stage for an incredible mistake that determined much of the course of science and religion. He believed in the 'burning log' assessment of the four natural elements. It was something that he could see. The log really did contain fire, air, water and earth. After the log was burned, the fire, air and water were gone – ascended into the heavens. The ashes, the earth, remained.

But animals were very different from logs, said Aristotle. They had to have a 'fifth essence' in their make-up. He called the stuff that gave life to animals 'quintessence', a term that survives to this day.

What kind of atom could make up 'quintessence'? There was only one choice, the one formed by pentagons, not triangles, the dodecahedron. Aristotle assigned this fifth atom the greatest nobility of any of the earthly atoms, a position that placed it above all the other atoms on earth and just below those of heaven. It linked man to the *primum mobile* that he believed to be at the edge of the spherical universe.

Aristotle was no armchair naturalist; he was an anatomist actively involved in animal dissections and was particularly interested in arteries and veins. He discovered that blood vessels in decapitated animals were especially hard to find and trace and elected to kill the animals he studied by the gruesome technique of strangulation. This made his dissections easier, but set the stage for his scientific error.

Aristotle's dissections had verified that there was a large rigid air tube that connected the mouth and nose to the lungs; this he named the 'trachea arteria', or the rough air tube. It is now called simply the trachea and is rough, or furrowed, since it is composed of many separate round rings of cartilage. Strangulation, he realized, blocked the trachea. The death that followed was proof that quintessence, which he sometimes called 'pneuma', was important to life. It was evidence, moreover, which supported his notion that man was linked by some kind of ether to the prime moving force in the heavens.

But Aristotle's insistence on killing animals by strangulation led him off the track. If animals are strangled, the pressure in the lungs eventually exceeds the pressure of the pumping right heart. Less blood can then flow through the lungs, and the left heart, in turn, receives less blood to push into arteries. Although the veins contain much more blood than is normal after strangulation, the arteries contain much less.

Thus Aristotle's careful dissections were done on animals that had overflowing veins and relatively empty arteries. When the arteries, which have a rigidity of their own, were opened by his scalpel, he found air and not much blood.

Many scientific historians have suggested that Aristotle's discovery of air in the arteries of dead animals was a colossal error in observation. This is not true. He observed something that most modern anatomists have missed. Although scientists cannot explain why, air *does* accumulate in arteries after animals die. This air accumulates in days, not hours, and does not develop in carcasses which are refrigerated or dissected soon after death. The best scientific evidence for this phenomenon is in dead human foetuses: the accumulation of air in the heart and arteries of the deceased foetus is so commonplace that it is used by doctors to confirm intrauterine death.

Aristotle began his experiments believing in four Platonic bodies, a spherical universe, a prime moving force, and a life-giving fifth essence. From his studies of strangulation, he concluded logically that quintessence, or pneuma, was carried from heaven through the trachea into the lungs and then into the heart. His subsequent discovery of hollow, air-filled tubes radiating from the heart led logically to the conclusion that pneuma flowed through these tubes to all organs of the body (see Fig. 5.1).

These conclusions led Aristotle to make an even larger mistake: he assigned the function of intelligent thought to the heart, not the brain. How could that happen? Aristotle was a student of plants, fish and animals and deeply interested in the hierarchy of creatures. He recognized that all these things were alive; they had a 'soul' that could pass out of them and lead to death. He concluded that a soul was a necessity for any living thing, then postulated a hierarchy of souls which matched his hierarchy of creatures.

Plants, the lowest form of life, had a vegetative soul that allowed them to grow and to reproduce. Animals, a higher form of life, had a vegetative soul for growth and reproduction, but they had an additional sensitive soul that allowed them to feel and to move. Man, the highest form of life, was capable of growth and reproduction, like a plant, and sensation and movement, like an animal. A vegetative and a sensitive soul allowed these activities. But man had a fifth ability: intelligent thought, which Aristotle believed came from the highest kind of soul, the rational soul.

This separation of souls, like many of Aristotle's other observations, would persist for centuries and would become incorporated in many Western religions.

If pneuma or quintessence was the fuel for rational thought, where was the organ of rational thought? There was only one logical place: in the heart. It not only received pneuma from the lungs, but also delivered it to the body through the air tubes.

Even though other people before and after Aristotle recognized that the brain was the seat of intelligence, his designation of the heart as the home of the highest soul and the organ of rational thought persisted for centuries. Many biblical scriptures speak of the heart as the organ of thought. 'Believe,' the Bible admonishes, 'with all thine heart.'

What did Aristotle think the brain did? Like Plato, he concluded that the brain was a gland. He believed it was a cooling gland that was placed in the head and near the nose for the purpose of regulating the temperature of the pneuma that was brought to it by the arteries.

Thus we see that both Plato and Aristotle conceived of the brain as a gland; both were correct, but for different and wrong reasons.

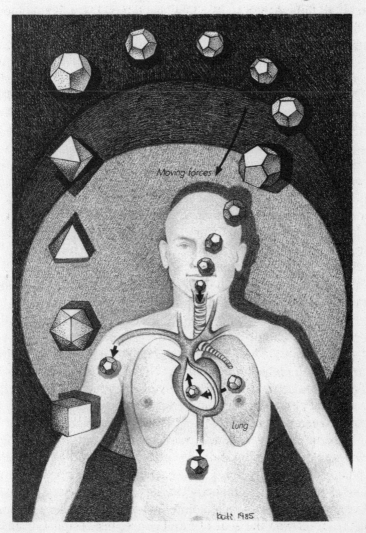

Fig. 5.1 Hollow arteries were central to Aristotle's belief that the heart was the organ of intelligent thought. He gave the dodecahedron a higher position than the other Platonic bodies and believed that it was pushed by a prime moving force in heaven into the body

A century later, Erasistratus (300–260 BC) described the nervous system in detail. Yet he held to Aristotle's notion that the rational soul resided in the heart. Finding three tubular structures going to every organ in the body – an artery, a vein and a nerve – Erasistratus postulated that pneuma was carried by the carotid arteries from the heart to the brain and flowed through nerves to all organs.

It was nearly 2,000 years before Aristotle's belief in the importance of quintessence was challenged. Although Galen found blood in arteries 550 years later, he still maintained that pneuma moved to and fro in arteries and supported Aristotle's notion that an ether-like substance descended from heaven into the arteries of man. It was the intellectual chicanery of Galen that ensured the longevity of this mismeme: he continued to support it even when he had made experimental observations that made it untenable. It was not until AD 1628, the year in which William Harvey published his classic book on the circulation of blood, that the belief in quintessence came into question.

Shoreline of Wonder

To understand the longevity of Aristotle's mismeme, we must recall the days when Aristotle served as the tutor to the teenager, Alexander. Aristotle's influence on Alexander was immense; years later Alexander would write: 'To my father I owe my life; to Aristotle the knowledge how to live it worthily.' During all his military campaigns Alexander slept with two things under his pillow: a dagger and a copy of Homer. Perhaps no other leader has held intellectual matters in such high regard.

As Alexander the Great moved along his route of conquest, he had taken with him the best engineers, surveyors, draftsmen and scribes from Greece. His reverence for rational thought and scholarship led him to insist that his conquering army preserve any material of academic interest. Thus, when they arrived in Egypt, they had in their possession not only the ideas of their conquered lands but also the scrolls and tablets that contained these ideas. In his well-planned fortified city a library was built that became the repository for this material.

Now you can see how the mismeme of Aristotle could so easily pass from the left brain of one scholar to the left brain of the next, and on for centuries. His great success with his student Alexander, his founding-father relationship with the Lyceum, his Macedonian birthplace, and his reverence for scholarship placed him at the hub of what might have been the first of the world's 'old boys' network', a complex amalgamation of privileged, educated, well-connected, financially secure and politically adroit men.

Inherent in any old boys' network is a belief that the members have special information-handling privileges. Whether in ancient Alexandria or modern institutional bureaucracies, an unnatural, divisive and inhuman conspiracy of silence comes to these kinds of organizations.

Can there be any doubt that the old Greeks' network in Alexandria or the old boys' networks in the schools, churches, and governments that followed are held together by the information in the left brain? Questions from the right brain can only disrupt the smooth-running of such places. In academic old boys' networks, those in command must use answers much as Mafia leaders use bullets.

Aristotle's error survived in large part because it assured the safe, central position of those in power in Alexandria. They had been selected for their ability to employ information in the defence of the besieged group and knew that Aristotle's paradigm was the strongest ammunition that existed. In that ancient academic place, as in most schools since, students gained admission by their ability to answer, not question. Socrates would not have passed the admission test for Alexandria; his incessant questions would have incensed the teachers there as much as they did his judges in Athens. Hunter would have been excluded from Alexandria because he had never been to primary school and couldn't read or write. And Leonardo? He would not have been allowed a second sheet of papyrus after his teachers had seen his mirror-writing.

In looking at Aristotle and the thinkers who preceded him, a pattern emerges: 'truths' are found by individuals, not institutions. They may be kept anywhere – in a cave, as those of Pythagoras were; or in a garden, as those of Plato were; or in a library, as those of Aristotle were. But always, when the truth-keepers accept para-digms that close out questions, or selfishly use answers as the bullets for their own defence, intellectual growth ceases.

6

Pagan in Saint's Clothing

Mount Everest was climbed, George Mallory said, because it was there. For centuries the mountain challenged men to make it to its peak, but during those attempts many unlucky climbers, including George Mallory, tumbled from its uncertain edges to their deaths. It is that way at the edge; some fall off.

On the next intellectual plateau, thinking people plunged, chained to each other, into the darkest intellectual abyss mankind has known. Their leader was Claudius Galen (AD 129–99).

In ancient Greece there were three kinds of medicine: that of Pythagoras, that of the Aesculapians, and that of Hippocrates. The Pythagorean medicine was based on mysticism; the Aesculapians believed in the healing power of snakes; and Hippocrates advocated a commonsense, nature-knows-best approach to medicine. By far the best organized system of medicine was that of the Aesculapians; they had more than 300 temples scattered throughout the world. Their largest centre was in Pergamon, the birthplace of Galen, who could not have escaped their influence; he remained an Aesculapian throughout his life.

At the age of fourteen Galen's medical studies began and by the age of twenty-one he felt he had outgrown his hometown teachers. He left for Corinth only to discover that his teacher had moved across the Mediterranean to the library at Alexandria. Galen followed him and remained a student in Alexandria until he was twenty-seven. In Alexandria he learned the medical lore, including the mismemes, of his honoured, ancient Greek forebears, Hippocrates and Aristotle.

After his medical education in Alexandria, Galen returned home and worked as the surgeon in the amphitheatre, aiding gladiators wounded by each other or by mauling lions. He, like many surgeons since, initially found his employment in treating victims of violence.

It is almost impossible to be long in an emergency medical situation and avoid the terror of an opened carotid artery. This is a most frightening sight. A patient's life blood may drain out before your eyes. Not ooze out, but spurt out – in seconds. Galen could not have been many days in the amphitheatre without witnessing a slit throat. It need only be seen once to realize that the carotid artery contains blood, not air.

Galen had learned his anatomy in Alexandria, where dissections were performed by slaves, but he constructed different laboratories, first in Pergamon and later in Rome, in which he did all his own dissections. Remarkably, these were performed in alive, awake animals. In his dissection room in Pergamon he performed the experiments which proved that his revered teachers, especially Aristotle, were wrong.

Galen may have been the first physician to take a patient-based observation to an animal laboratory. His experiment is well described in one of his many books. In a living animal he exposed an artery in the groin and tied a ligature around it. Beyond the point of ligation, the artery stopped pulsating. There he opened the artery and placed a hollow quill into it. He secured the quill within the lumen of the artery with a second ligature, then released the first. No air came out of the now-pulsatile artery, only blood.

By this first surgical experiment Galen proved that Aristotle was wrong; blood, not air, was flowing through arteries. With this single observation Galen could have challenged Aristotle's paradigm that thoughts are pneumatic and done what none of his Alexandrian teachers had been able to do: bring science back to a commitment to questions rather than answers.

Galen connected his new-found information about blood in arteries to the paradigm chain that linked Pythagoras, Empedocles, Plato, Aristotle, Hippocrates, Erasistratus and all of those at Alexandria. To make it fit, the other paradigms that Galen revered needed very little modification. But Galen must have known that without pneuma in arteries, nearly everything that Aristotle had taught about the nature of man, indeed the nature of the world, would come into question.

Galen at this pivotal moment elected to construct his own paradigm and used each paradigm of the ancient Greeks to buttress his notions. With little modification he accepted the atoms with triangular skin of the Pythagoreans, the fire/earth/water/air elements of Empedocles, the perfectly spherical divine universe of Plato, the prime moving force of the universe of Aristotle, the vegetable, animal and rational souls of Aristotle, the quintessence of Aristotle, the four humours of Empedocles and Hippocrates and the notion of Erasistratus that nerves are hollow tubes which carry quintessence from the brain.

Aristotle had employed the notion of 'hollow arteries' as a central concept upon which he skewered several unrelated paradigms. Galen's discovery of blood in the carotids could have been the antidote to that pernicious mismeme.

Galen, however, performed a feat of intellectual legerdemain in forming a compromise between new facts and old myths. He contended that arterial blood was intermixed with the quintessence of Aristotle – that both were carried in arteries – and by that maintained the viability of Aristotle's mismeme.

Galen was quick to recognize that the blood that he found in arteries was very different from that in veins; it was bright red, rather than dark red, and didn't drain out, but was forcibly pushed from an open vessel.

Arterial blood is not easily obtained, even today. The arteries of the body are generally hidden deep in the centre of the abdomen, arm, or leg, but the veins are quite superficial.

Needles and syringes were not invented until the American civil war in 1865 and before that time those who wished to drain blood from a human or an animal resorted to 'cupping'. In this procedure a cup was held under an open vessel, typically opened with a scalpel or lance, and blood was allowed to flow into the cup. Since cupping was a superficial procedure, it drained blood from veins, not arteries.

Once in a cup blood coagulates, and then separates into a dark purple clot at the bottom and an overlying pool of yellow serum. Most often, the clot is visibly covered with a thin layer of white material. No doubt this had been observed for centuries before three substances mixed together. In the amphitheatre or in the animal laboratory, Galen must have witnessed this separation of blood.

Until the experiments of Galen proved there was blood in the carotid arteries, there was no need to consider the make-up of arterial blood. But lacking syringes, even though Galen knew that arteries contained blood, it was technically difficult to collect such blood and compare it to venous blood.

Galen's study of blood gained him everlasting fame: he said that blood contained four different kinds of humours – just as the burning log was composed of four different Platonic bodies. He concluded that venous blood was a mixture of three humours: black bile, yellow bile and phlegm. The clot that he saw was the black bile, the serum was the yellow bile, and the white material that separated clot from serum was the phlegm. Arterial blood was made of different stuff. It was bright red and driven with such force from the artery that it was not easily collected into a cup for analysis. This was pure blood – sanguine.

Although Galen could see only four humours in blood, he held to Aristotle's concept that quintessence was carried from the heavens into the lungs, through the heart and into the arteries. Moreover, he went further. He postulated that pneuma entered the body in two places: through the lungs and the pores of the skin. The pulsation of sanguine within arteries, he contended, came from the rhythmical entrance of pneuma into arteries, first into the lungs and then into the pores. It was pneuma that gave life to the arteries, not the pulsating heart. It was pneuma that entered the lung and pushed arterial blood out of the chest; it was pneuma that entered the pores of the skin and the 'mouths' of the arteries to push arterial blood back into the chest. This to-and-fro movement of blood came entirely from pneuma; the heart was not involved (see Fig. 6.1).

Sanguine was Galen's discovery. He could put it wherever he wanted to put it (in arteries), assign whatever behavioural qualities to it he wished (goodness), and allow it to co-mingle with Aristotle's arterial quintessence.

Galen could rewrite history according to his own views, and he rewrote it very clearly:

In the universe there are four elements – fire, air, water, and earth; and in the living body there are four humours, black bile, yellow bile, sanguine, and phlegm. Out of the excess or deficiency or misproportion of these four humours there arise disease; by restoring the correct proportion diseases are cured.

For the next fifteen centuries barber surgeons would employ scalpels, cups or leeches to drain patients of their bad humours. Alchemists, predecessors to modern physicians, during this period used the same paradigm to design their herbal and magical treatments.

Medicine, philosophy and religion became imbued with Galen's view that humours linked people to their worlds, indeed, controlled their minds and 'souls'. To Galen, and to the priests and philosophers who heeded him, the mysterious soul was of far greater importance than the mind.

Galen had accepted Aristotle's view of a vegetative, an animal and a rational soul. But he was more specific; he took the three largest solid organs in the body – the liver, the heart, and the brain – to be the anatomical homes for these three souls.

Venous blood, Galen thought, was formed in the liver and propelled by the force of the vegetative soul through the body's veins. This view of the liver was accepted for centuries. It is

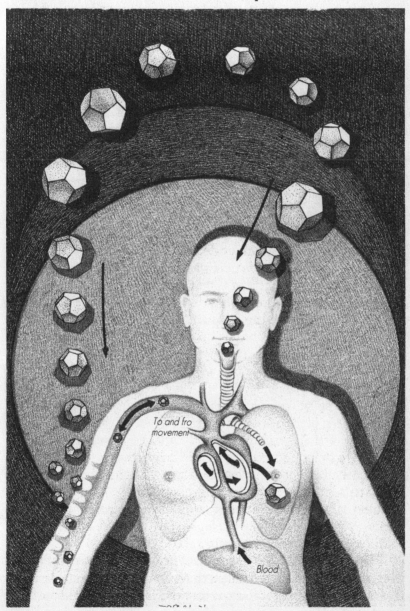

Fig. 6.1 Galen discovered that arteries were filled with blood, not air, but maintained his belief in Aristotle's quintessence. He assumed quintessence entered arterial pores and caused the to-and-fro movement of blood

reflected in the anatomical drawings of the sixteenth-century anatomist Andrea Vesalius (AD 1514–64).

Galen viewed the heart as a mixing place, where some venous blood could pass through 'pores' into the arterial blood, where the 'sooty stuff' could pass out of veins through the heart and out the lungs, where heat could be added to the venous and arterial blood that moved in and out, and where pneuma could be added to arterial blood. But what was most important, the heart housed an animal soul that generated heat and movement.

Galen believed that the best soul, the rational soul, resided in the brain and in that belief was the first of all the ancient Greeks to link the brain to intelligent thought. To each soul Galen assigned a spirit. 'Natural' spirit came to the body through the liver, 'vital' spirit came in through the heart, and 'animal' spirit was added by the brain. His views of animal spirit are especially important to the history of brain science, for what he preached remained a central dogma until the Renaissance. Animal spirit was the stuff of thought.

Erasistratus, five centuries before Galen, had discovered the nervous system that Aristotle had overlooked. Erasistratus claimed that Aristotle's pneuma was carried by hollow nerves from the brain to all other organs. Galen accepted this and, as surely as he maintained a place for pneuma in hollow arteries, he maintained a place for pneuma in the hollow brain; he believed that pneuma was transformed by the brain into animal spirit, which in turn was carried through the tubular nerves to the body.

Galen extended the importance of animal spirit to muscles. Noting that muscles bulged when they contracted, he postulated that animal spirit, released from nerve ends into muscles, caused the muscle to puff up and contract. This mechanistic view of brain and nerve activity was maintained until the eighteenth century; Fig. 6.2, a drawing from AD 1739, shows such mysterious stuff being pushed out of the spinal cord of a frog to make the muscles contract.

Galen did with the four humours of the blood what Empedocles, Plato and Aristotle did with the four elements of the burning log: he assigned goodness or badness to each of them.

Galen was very positive about sanguine, the humour that flowed in arteries, and reasoned that those who were blessed with a rich supply were directed, robust and strong, much like arterial blood itself.

To black bile, which he called 'melancholy', he assigned the negative quality of sadness. It was this stuff he believed that led to

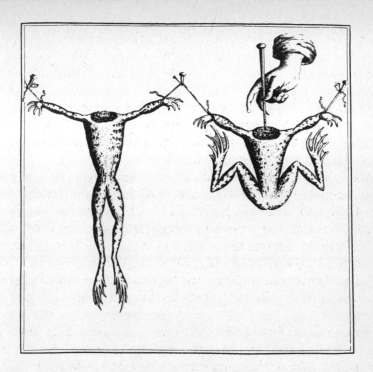

Fig. 6.2 'Animal spirit' is pushed out of the spinal cord of a frog to make the frog's muscles contract, according to Galen

melancholic depression. This term has been linked to that kind of behaviour ever since.

To yellow bile, 'choler', Galen assigned the negative qualities of bitterness and anger. Ever since, hot-tempered irascible people have been described as choleric.

To 'phlegm' he assigned the negative qualities of dull, sluggish inactivity and ever since people with that kind of behaviour have been called phlegmatic.

All three of the old humours are bad humours; only one good humour existed – the stuff that Galen had discovered in arteries.

The third venous humour, 'phlegm', was of most concern to Galen, a practising physician. Sadness and anger, the result of the first two humours, were both tolerable and not causes of disease, he reasoned. But an accumulation of phlegm, he believed, could disrupt the body's functions. Galen, a good observer, might have noted an excess of phlegm in his patients who were ill and might have reasoned that it was the cause of the disease, not the result. To this day, the quantitative measurement of the white layer found between the red cells and the serum of clotted blood is employed to diagnose infections of many types, for this layer is none other than white cells, the scavenger cells that accumulate within the blood during infection.

The presence of excessive phlegm in the blood, coupled to the notion that this was the cause of phlegmatic behaviour, led Galen to push for 'cupping' in patients who were sick to the point of sluggishness. In modern times some of the best of men, George Washington, and the worst men, Adolph Hitler, have been cupped; Washington with lances and Hitler with leeches.

Galen saw a unique safety valve attached to the brain that could remove its excessive phlegm and thus cleanse the rational soul. This was the pituitary gland. 'Pituita' is an ancient colloquial word for the mucus that accumulates in or runs from the nose: 'snot'. Galen believed that pituita came from the pituitary gland, not the nose, and reasoned that during illness it was drained from the brain through the pituitary into the nose. In that day, as in this, excessive secretions from the nose and throat are commonly seen in infectious diseases. Thus Galen may have observed very sick, phlegmatic patients draining 'pituita' from the airway and, given his starting point, this would have been a logical deduction.

Galen's view of the pituitary emphasizes the lengths that he would go to support his paradigm that thoughts are 'humoural'. Although he was a careful anatomist and skilled at dissection, he postulated many unseen anatomical structures whenever his fiction needed physical support. He described 'mouths' in arteries near the skin through which pneuma could flow and 'pores' in the septum of the heart through which the 'sooty stuff' of venous blood could pass; and he wrote about bone perforations beneath the pituitary that allowed 'phlegm' to reach the nose. Arteries do not have 'mouths', the septum of the heart does not have 'pores', and the skull beneath the pituitary has no perforations. Galen wrote 22,000 pages of descriptive anatomy; he was no amateur anatomist. Yet to serve his paradigm he literally poked the body full of holes that didn't exist.

By bending the 'truth' only slightly, Galen was able to keep the ancient Greek paradigms secure, and his own paradigm became central to all the others.

Chemists were pleased. By his four humours, the four elements – fire, air, earth, and water – were validated and with them teachers could continue to teach about the four Platonic bodies in the burning log.

Philosophers were pleased. Including pneuma in arteries and in the brain and nerves allowed teachers to espouse Aristotle's belief that quintessence linked man to his maker.

Theologians were pleased. Stressing the importance of 'souls' as propelling forces for blood preserved the priest's high regard for an ethereal soul.

Astrologers were pleased. The perfectly spherical universe with perfect circular movement of the heavenly bodies was left undisturbed by his to–and–fro movement of blood in arteries and veins.

Physicians were pleased. The medical belief of Hippocrates that humours were important causative agents of disease was not only supported but also extended.

By keeping Aristotle's pneuma in arteries, sanguine was allowed to mix with the most noble of all elements: quintessence. By his paradigm that thoughts are 'humoural' he had explained the earthly elements, the body, the soul and the mind.

Galen's mismeme kept the old Greeks' network together. It survived as the 'truth' from AD 160 until AD 1628, the year that William Harvey convinced the world that blood was not driven to and fro by 'souls', as Galen had preached.

Shoreline of Wonder

Galen's paradigm for brain function, like all ancient and all modern paradigms, involved 'scientific reductionism'. The complexities of the mind were reduced to elements that could be described in words and numbers and then passed from teacher to student.

All the reductions preceding Galen had maintained the view that the brain was a gland. Plato thought that it secreted semen. Aristotle concluded it was a cooling gland. Erasistratus thought it pushed fluid down hollow nerves.

Galen's concept of the brain was the best formed, for his paradigm allowed some secretions to come to the brain and allowed other secretions to drain from the brain. Central to his paradigm was the reduction of both physical and mental diseases to simple causes, humours, which could be dealt with by simple techniques. The therapy that he popularized, cupping, was so simple that even the untutored could do it.

Both the Christian and the Islamic religions helped to ensure the passage of Galen's mismeme for seventy generations. Both religions maintained that Galen had given the world the 'truth' about the body; it was written in his words, and pictures were not needed. In their rejection of pictures, the priests and scribes, the 'keepers of the truth', did what Empedocles had done with the wisdom of Pythagoras: they excluded the right brain, which serves dually as the creator of pattern-dependent paradigms and the verifier of paradigm reliability. It was this exclusion that allowed Galen's mismeme to pass, without challenge or change, for such a long period.

By his anatomical studies and his knowledge of blood-filled arteries, Galen was within an ace of discovering the circulation of the blood. But imbued by the ancient Greek notion that only the stars could move in circles, he assigned blood a to-and-fro movement.

The consequence of this intellectual compromise was immense: it left Aristotle unscathed and allowed the belief in the 'nobility of the elements' to remain in place.

If Richard Dawkins is correct in saying that genes are only body shapers, that memes shape civilization, then certainly we must look about for some mismeme that entered the minds of people and mis-shaped civilization during the dark ages. No wrong paradigm of that era compares to that of Galen; it was of the appropriate elements, in the right place, at the right time and supported by the right institutions. Galen, by my measure, can not escape blame.

Galen was a pagan and, certainly, he did not support the Roman church. That a pagan's written words became religious foundation stones is one of history's greatest ironies.

7

One Picture is Worth a Thousand Years

A ndrea Vesalius (AD 1514–64) may have been mute because he used few words to lead mankind out of the quagmire of Galenic humours. His pictures, published in AD 1543, in his book, *The Fabric of Man*, speak for themselves.

Few published documents have challenged as many major issues at once as *The Fabric of Man*. It was obvious from the frontispiece (Fig. 7.1) that Vesalius was 'desecrating' the human body. He presented not only the bare skin of man but also bare muscles, nerves, blood vessels and bones.

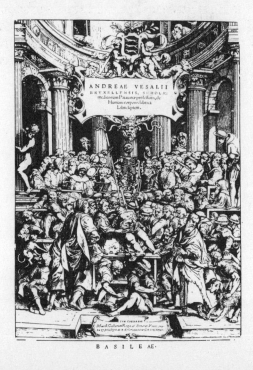

Fig. 7.1 The frontispiece of Vesalius's *The Fabric of Man*

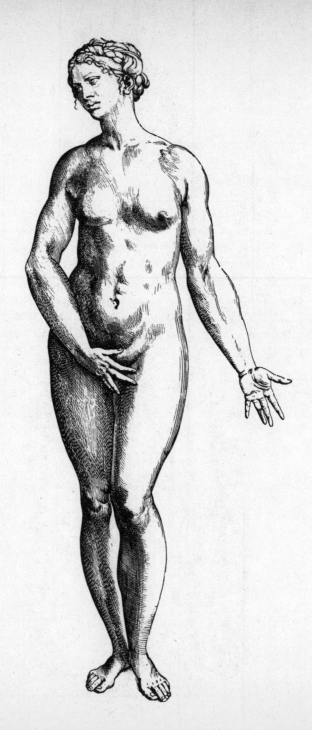

Fig. 7.2 Vesalius's nude female

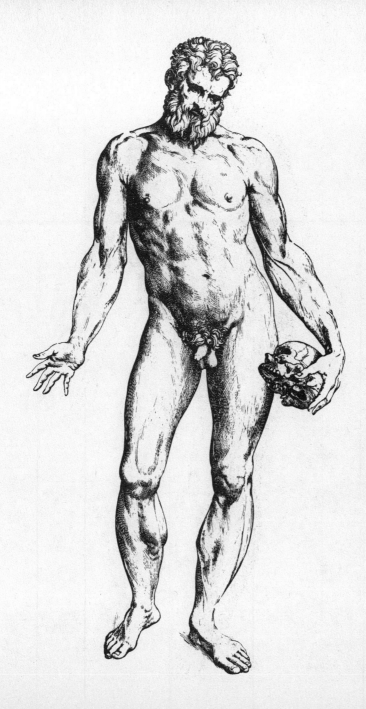

Fig. 7.3 Vesalius's nude male

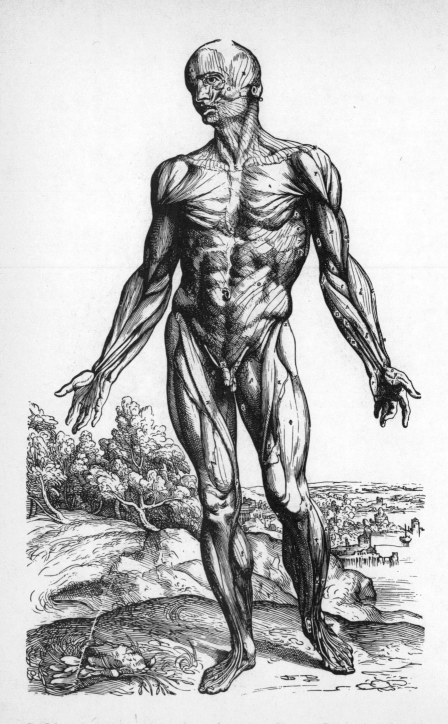

Fig. 7.4 Vesalius's skinless male

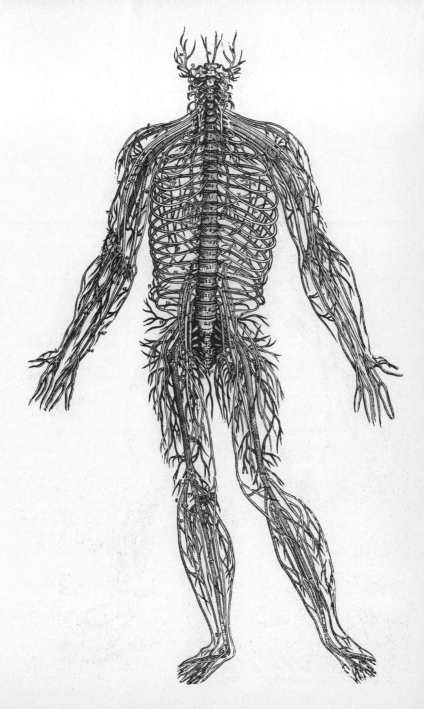

Fig. 7.5 Vesalius on nerves of the body

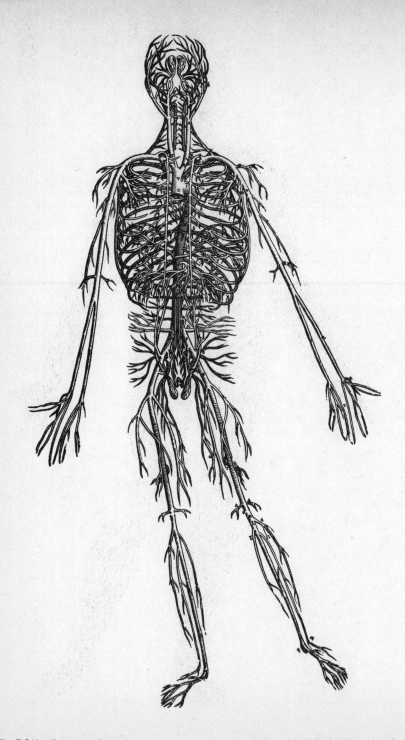

Fig. 7.6 Vesalius on arteries

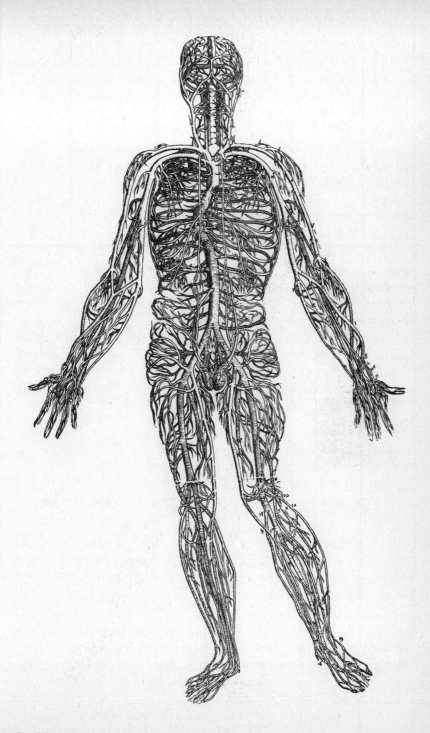

Fig. 7.7 Vesalius on veins

The series of pictures (Figs 7.2–7.7) freed people's minds from the chains of Galen's paradigm. These pictures were published ten years before Michael Servetus was burned at the stake for claiming that blood 'circulates' from the heart to the lungs and back to the heart. The church was still very much in power, controlling not only the writers' pens but also the painters' brushes, still contending that bodies should not be dissected, and still preaching the infallibility of Galen.

Until the publication of *The Fabric of Man*, the reverence that was given to the skin and flesh of the human body foreclosed any questions about it; without such questions there could be no biological progress. Every drawing that Vesalius did of 'form' presaged a question concerning 'function'; his anatomy book became the guiding chart for the physiological books that would follow. As Vesalius stripped the skin and the flesh from the body, he broke apart the chain of answers that Galen had wrapped around people's minds. Questions about the validity of Galen's written words, the Platonic bodies of Empedocles, the spherical universe of Plato and Aristotle's prime moving force were now mandatory.

Seventy-three years after the publication of *The Fabric of Man*, Galen was dethroned: on 17 April 1616, William Harvey announced in London that blood did not move to and fro in arteries and veins as Galen taught. It circulated.

Harvey's discovery can be traced back to Vesalius, who wrote in AD 1555:

Not long ago I would not have dared to diverge a hair's breadth from Galen's opinion. But the septum of the heart is as thick, dense and compact as the rest of the heart. I do not see, therefore, how even the smallest particle can be transferred from the right to the left ventricle through it.

Harvey studied in Padua in AD 1603 with the academic successors of Vesalius and learned then that Galen's paradigm was no longer accepted. He returned to London and performed experiments initially in sheep but later in forty other animal species to prove the observation of Vesalius. He cut away a portion of the beating heart and showed that no blood came through the septum. By mathematical calculations, he verified that the volume of blood passing through the heart in an hour was far greater than the weight of the entire animal; proof that blood was circulating.

Harvey did not publish his immortal book, *On the Motion of the Heart and Blood*, until AD 1628, twelve years after his discovery. There, Harvey wrote:

Since calculations and visual demonstrations have confirmed all my suppo-sitions, to wit, that the blood is passed through the lungs and the heart by the pulsation of the ventricles, is forcibly ejected to all parts of the body, therein steals into the veins and porosities of the flesh, flows back everywhere through those very veins from the circumference to the centre, from small veins into larger ones, and thence comes at last into the vena cava and to the auricle of the heart; I am obliged to conclude that in animals the blood is driven round a circuit with an unceasing, circular sort of movement, that this is an activity or function of the heart which it carries out by virtue of its pulsation, and that in sum it constitutes the sole reason for the heart's pulsatile movement.

To buttress his arguments about circulation Harvey included the drawing shown in Fig. 7.8.

One of Vesalius's pictures, shown in Fig. 7.9, stands apart. It subtly describes the predicament of thinking people, then and now. Vesalius has positioned the bones between a precipice and a judge's table – between the uncertain edge and the certain solid centre – and then thrown a skull on the judge's table. He has drawn the lonely bones, stripped of everything, between the centre and the edge, not only pondering the skull but fondling it, right under the nose of the authorities who had said to him that neither ques-tions, nor drawings, nor dissections were permitted. It is a self-portrait. In this drawing, Vesalius has challenged those at the centre to either accept his questions, dissections, drawings – his desecrations – or push him off the edge.

Shoreline of Wonder

The term 'lateral thinking' comes from a book by that name writ-ten some years ago by Edward De Bono. In it he describes the kind of intellectual end-runs that the human mind can make around the problems and puzzles it faces. It is the quality that cannot be taught; some people are better at it than others.

I have seen a special kind of 'lateral thinking' in the ascending brains of students and in the descending brains of those who are ill. Being with those who are very sick has allowed me to watch hundreds of face-to-face encounters between the human mind and its problems. Countless times I have watched my patients twist

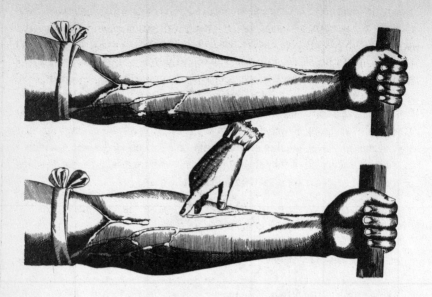

Fig. 7.8 Harvey's drawing to show one-way venous valves. This simple observation proved that venous blood moved towards the heart

their problems into opportunities: I have seen average students become superior students when they became paraplegic, those with night-time pain rise to write, and the threat of headache drive many to near-perfect performances. As a bystander it appears to me that the human mind, in its darkest hours, seeks the brightest guiding star. It seems to thrive on the conversion of problems to opportunities.

If you think about the mirror-writing of Leonardo, the dyslexia of John Hunter, or, in more modern times, the blindness of Helen Keller, the paraplegia of Franklin Roosevelt, or the discrimination against Gandhi and Martin Luther King, you have to ask, 'What drives the minds that convert their problems to opportunities?'

The magnificent accomplishments of each suggests there is a mental force that wells up from their most tragic flaw. Somehow these people are able to draw on a force that provides inner healing and overflows in a creative force that heals the world around them. Does the magic of their lives spring from the more harmonious use of the right and left brain? I doubt it.

What is it and where does it come from? I have come to believe that from some deep recess in the right brain springs a 'sense of beauty', perhaps the human mind's highest intellectual ability. The great individuals of the past – Leonardo, Vesalius, Hunter – and Keller, Roosevelt, Gandhi, King – my modern role models, the best students I have taught, and those who have coped most successfully with their illnesses have all been imbued with a sense of beauty. This may be the mind's 'black hole': a hidden star that is only seen when all around is totally without light.

It was the pattern-dependent sense of beauty in the right brain of Vesalius that led humankind out of the dark ages.

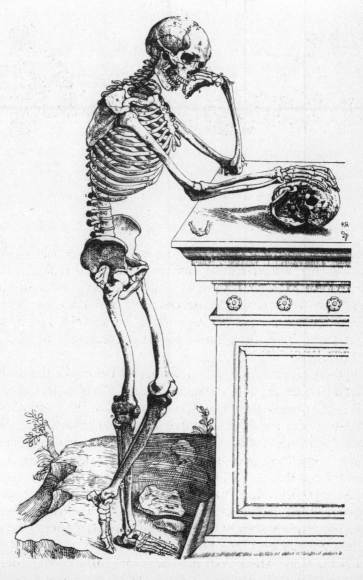

Fig. 7.9 A self-portrait of Vesalius? The lonely figure stands at the edge of a cliff, figuratively asking those in authority to accept his dissections or push him off the edge

8

The Understanding of Brain Electricity

*T*he burning log was important to the thoughts of all ancient philosophers and scientists. The four Platonic bodies were basic to their understanding of the heavens, the earth, the sea, animal and plant life, and the body, soul and mind of man.

Modern physicists believe that the burning log is composed of four separate forces: a strong nuclear force, which holds together the big pieces of the atomic nucleus, a weak nuclear force, which influences the little pieces of atoms, gravity, which pulls things towards the central mass point of the earth, and an electromagnetic force, which permeates all matter.

Although no one has seen any of these four forces, the brightest among us – the modern day Platos – insist that they exist. Moreover, scientists are convinced that there is a fifth force that unites and drives the other four. Einstein, like most great physicists, went to his grave trying to prove a 'unified field theory' that would bring the other four forces together.

The belief that electricity, the fourth of the modern forces, is the stuff of thought has permeated brain science since the late 1700s. Yet this has led to a deep schism between brain scientists and other biologists; while the brain was regarded as 'dry', all other organs were conceived of as 'wet'. Doubtless the study of brain electricity helped in the understanding of the internal circuits of the brain, but it solved few problems of brain disease.

Our next intellectual ascent will trace the step-by-step developments that led to the belief that the brain was driven by electricity. Each of the guides for this ascent introduced a new paradigm, and in each case the new discovery was an outgrowth of a previous paradigm. At the bottom is Benjamin Franklin; at the top is Egas Moniz:

1940   Egas Moniz (pre-frontal lobotomy)
1936   Herb Gasser (electrical nerve impulse)
1934   Henry Dale (chemical neurotransmission)
1906   Charles Sherrington (synaptic function)
1900   Ramon y Cajal (nerve synapses)
1890   Sigmund Freud (fundamental psychiatry)
1890   Hughlings Jackson (fundamental neurology)
1890   Victor Horsley (fundamental neurosurgery)
1885   Camillo Golgi (nerve histology)
1856   Claude Bernard (neural networks)
1839   Theodore Schwann (animal cells)
1792   Luigi Galvani (animal electricity)
1753   Benjamin Franklin (electricity)

Ben Franklin's creative genius extended to publishing, politics, finance, insurance, statesmanship, machinery, writing, optics, heating and science. Ben Franklin, the electrician, had often participated in 'parlor trick' experiments that used the Leiden jar, a Dutch invention. By rapidly rotating a sulfur ball inside an insulated glass container, a current of electricity was generated which could reverse magnets, melt metal, create an audible explosion and even kill some animals.

On a rainy day in Philadelphia in 1752, Ben Franklin performed some momentous outdoor experiments. Certainly aware of the risk, Franklin flew a kite into a thunder cloud. By attaching one of the kite strings to a Leiden jar, he was able to 'trap' the electrical forces of the heavens in the earth-bound vessel. In doing this he verified that the swirling raindrops in the thundercloud and the rotating sulfur ball in the Leiden jar were producing the same kind of electricity. He knew instantly that all matter and all animals were linked to the heavens by this mysterious stuff.

The parallel between Aristotle's pneuma and Franklin's electricity is glaring. Aristotle postulated a paradigm that carried unseen stuff – pneuma – into the soul of man. Franklin postulated another kind of unseen stuff that was carried into the body of man. Pneuma was assigned a life-giving goodness, yet it carried mankind down a wrong-way non-productive intellectual path for 2,000 years. Electricity had a life-threatening badness about it, yet it has steered scientists along their most fertile intellectual path.

The following discoveries all sprang from Ben Franklin's rainy-day experiment: Galvani's understanding of animal electricity, Volta's development of the voltaic cell – the battery, Oerstad's development of the electromagnetic motor, Faraday's development of the electricity-producing dynamo, Faraday's marriage of light waves and electromagnetic waves, Maxwell's electromagnetic wave-form equations, Hertz's production of electromagnetic waves, Morse's development of the telegraph, Bell's development of the telephone, Marconi's development of radio, Edison's development of the incandescent light, Edison's development of the phonograph, Zworkin's development of television, Neumann's development of the computer and Shockley's development of the transistor.

Geniuses such as Franklin have the ability to ask questions that have a transparent quality; they can look out of themselves and see substance in a thing that everyone else looks through as if it were not there. All of the greatest intellectual advances of science grow from such transparent questions. Franklin was not the first to see the Leiden jar, a lightning bolt or a kite, but he saw the connecting issue. He gave substance to the issue by asking, 'Could an unseen electrical force extend through our universe?' The spark of genius was not in the experiment or even in the tools of the experiment; it was in the transparent question that started it all.

Luigi Galvani (1737–98), an Italian anatomist, discovered animal electricity. He was educated to believe that animal spirit flowed through nerves. An anatomist, doubtless he had seen the drawing of the beheaded frog on page 43 and had read this statement by Rene Descartes (1596–1660):

The cavities of the brain are central reservoirs ... animal spirits enter these cavities. They pass into the pores of its substance and from these pores into the nerves. The nerves may be compared to the tubes of a waterworks; breathing or other actions depend upon the flow of animal spirits into the nerves. The rational soul (the pineal) takes the place of the engineer, *living* in that part of the reservoir that connects all of the various tubes. These spirits are like the wind. When they flow into a muscle they cause it to become stiff and harden, just as air in a balloon makes it hard.

Most probably, Galvani had also compared the drawings of the ventricle of his countryman, Vesalius, to those of Descartes (see Fig. 8.1).

In the centuries between Galen and Descartes, the best thinkers believed that muscles contracted because they were puffed up by brain fluid, or animal spirit, which was transported to them by hollow nerves. Thus the view that thoughts are driven by water was a scientific fact in AD 1791, the year that Galvani discovered animal electricity.

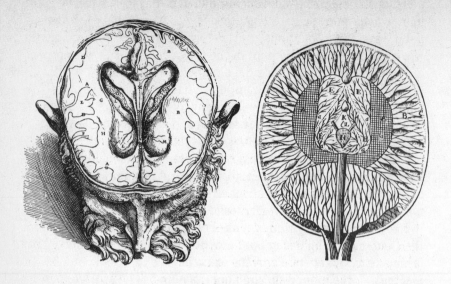

Fig. 8.1 Vesalius (left) and Descartes (right) believed, as Galen did, that fluid was stored in the ventricles of the brain before it was pushed down hollow nerves into muscles

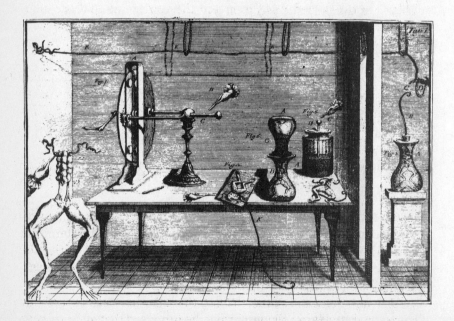

Fig. 8.2 Galvani used many different kinds of electrical stimuli to show that electricity caused muscles to contract

Galvani described the discovery like this:

Prepared frogs, which were fastened by brass hooks in their spinal cord to an iron railing which surrounded a certain hanging garden of my home, fell into contractions not only when lightning flashed, but even when the sky was quiet . . . I began to press the brass hooks upon the iron railing . . . and . . . I observed frequent contractions which had no relation to the changes in the electrical state of the atmosphere.

Once he had made these initial observations, Galvani was able to take electricity from a variety of sources and produce twitching in frog legs (see Fig. 8.2). In making these observations Galvani destroyed a paradigm that had survived for 2,200 years.

Initially Galvani's observation was greeted with enthusiasm by his colleagues. They shared his belief that the frog, like the torpedo fish, contained electricity, and they accepted his view that this, not animal spirit, controlled muscular activity.

Perhaps the most visible of his early supporters was Allessandro Volta (1745–1827), a fellow Italian. But Volta's support was short-lived; he repeated the experiments and verified that the twitching only happened if the metals employed were dissimilar. In doing that he challenged Galvani's notion that the frog itself produced electricity; to Volta the frog muscle was only storing electricity. This controversy led Volta to invent the voltaic cell that produces electricity by the interactions of certain metals and other acids; the batteries that are important to your daily life sprang from the argument that went on between Galvani and Volta.

Despite his critics, Galvani stuck to his belief that the response to an external electrical stimulus could only mean that a similar stimulus within the animal itself forced muscles to contract. This has been confirmed millions of times since 1792, in all kinds of animals including people.

Again we see the power of the paradigm: one man looked at one string – this time threaded through frog legs. What he saw changed the world.

Theodore Schwann (1810–82) was a brilliant anatomist who first described animal cells. Convinced by those around him that the brain was driven by animal electricity, he made a mistake at the very beginning of brain studies that matches the 'hollow arteries' of Aristotle and the 'four humours' of Galen.

Although Schwann acknowledged that all other cells in the body were separated by a cell membrane, he proposed that all brain cells were united in a giant network that carried Galvani's brain electricity. He strongly denied the bridging points between nerves that we now call 'synapses', and his stature as the world's senior brain anatomist cemented that erroneous view in place for seven decades.

Schwann's discoveries depended upon improved microscopes and the development of microtomes – the laboratory devices that cut tissue into ultra-thin slices. Thomas Kuhn, in *The Structure of Scientific Revolutions*, observed that most new paradigms spring from technological advances, and the discovery of animal cells is a classic example of creative thought's technological dependency.

A London physician, Robert Brown, first employed the microscope in 1831 to observe the nucleus of the plant cell. Using better equipment, Mathius Schleiden (1804–81) in 1838 found a clearly defined cell membrane around each plant cell nucleus. Schleiden said that each cell was like an egg; it contained a central nucleus similar to the yolk, a surrounding cytoplasm similar to egg-white and an outer membrane like the egg shell. All plants, he said, were bundles of separate cells, and each cell had a 'life' of its own; the life of the plant came from the symbiotic working-together of many different kinds of cells.

Theodore Schwann, working in Louvain, was quick to employ the microtome and better microscopes to see the same thing in animals. In 1839 Schwann proposed that animals, like plants, were aggregates of individual membrane-bound cells. His friend, Rudolph Virchow (1821–1902) in Berlin, taught a generation of pathologists and other physicians about the importance of cells to disease and, in 1858, wrote:

Every animal is a sum of vital units, each of which possesses the full characteristics of life. The character and unity of life cannot be found in one definite point of higher organization, for example, in the brain of man, but only in the definite, constantly recurring disposition shown individually by each single element. It follows that the composition of the major organism, the so-called individual, must be likened to a kind of social arrangement or society, in which a number of separate existencies are dependent upon one another, in such a way, however, that each element possesses its own peculiar activity and carries out its own task by its own powers.

Schwann accepted this description of animal cells and taught that organs were composed of individual cells living in symbiosis. Each cell was totally enveloped by its cell membrane. But he argued that brain cells needed to know what their neighbours were doing; they could not have private envelopes that fenced them off from other cells. He proposed that the brain was composed of a giant network of cells, a three-dimensional spider web composed of millions of threads, but that in this web every nerve cell was directly connected to every other nerve cell (see Fig. 8.3).

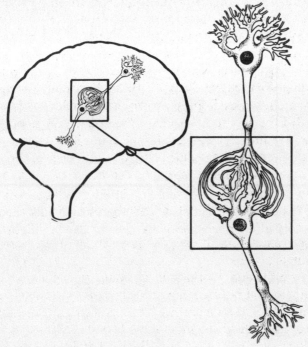

Fig. 8.3 Schwann's view of nerve connections

He was led to this erroneous position by the limitation of his microscope for he could not, with his techniques, see the synapses that we now know connect one nerve to another. But as certainly as Aristotle's belief in 'quintessence' led to his ready acceptance of hollow arteries, a belief in Galvani's brain electricity led Schwann to accept the notion that a giant circuit of cell wires united the brain; without a 'circuit', electricity could not flow through the brain.

It was Ramon y Cajal who discovered synapses in 1900, but the father of cellular anatomy, Theodore Schwann, and the father of cellular pathology, Rudolph Virchow, both adhered to the network theory of brain cells. More important, perhaps, was the acceptance of this theory by Claude Bernard (1813–78), the Parisian father of physiology. Bernard kept a little red notebook by his bedside and would write in it random night-time thoughts. In 1856 we find these words written in Bernard's notebook: 'Consider the brain to be a gland; put catheters in the veins of the brain and stimulate the sympathetic nerves.' His daytime teachings were very different. Although he urged scientists of all kinds to study the 'internal milieu' of the body, he accepted Schwann's dictum that the cells of the brain were wired together in a way that made the internal milieu superfluous to neuronal activity.

During this period, patient care strategies and educational programmes in psychiatry, neurology and neurosurgery were being developed. The founding father of each of these disciplines – Sigmund Freud (1856–1939) in psychiatry, Hughlings Jackson (1835–1911) in neurology and Victor Horsley (1857–1916) in neurosurgery – were all infected with Schwann's mismeme. The early respect that psychiatry, neurology and neurosurgery gave to Schwann's wrong view of the brain has warped the development of each of these branches of medicine.

Very few physicians now caring for patients with brain illnesses are aware that their specialty was rooted in such shaky sand: only now, a century after this lamentable mistake, are brain physicians aware that brain cells are in every way like all other cells in the body.

Perhaps no other name has been so inextricably woven into the language of the brain as Schwann's. Schwann cells are often the first cells that are described to young medical students and, for whatever reason, long after all other neuroanatomical facts are forgotten, physicians of all kinds still remember these nerve cells and can describe them in detail. Schwann was correct about most cellular matters but wrong about brain cells; this has a special kind of historical irony. A Schwann cell is illustrated in Fig. 8.4.

In the past decade it has become obvious that the secrets of the brain will only be understood by looking inside the cell, not at the electricity that flows along the surface of the cell. Thus, not for his network theory and not for the cells that bear his name, but for his fundamental contributions to biology, all brain scientists are in debt to Schwann.

In their natural state, cells have a very transparent quality – they resemble jellyfish – and only by staining them with a dye can their details be seen. The dyes that are used by anatomists to paint or stain the cell are numerous and each cell, indeed, each part of every cell, can be stained with a different dye.

In 1871 the network theory of nerves was given a tremendous boost by the development of a new method of staining brain cells. Camillo Golgi (1843–1926) discovered that silver salts, which would bind to the surface of the nerves and nowhere else, could be added to brain tissue. Why this should be remains a biochemical

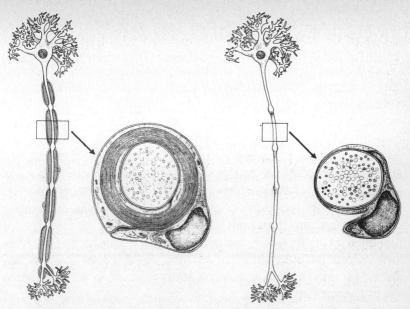

Fig. 8.4 A schwann cell with its jelly-like myelin wrapper (left) and a nerve without myelin (right)

mystery, but the pictures that Golgi presented to the world were things of beauty.

Golgi's photographs seemed to confirm that a giant spider web united the nerves of the nervous system. But at the end of that century a quiet Spaniard, Santiago Ramon y Cajal, employed the same stains that Golgi had used to demonstrate something startlingly different. Cajal noted that every nerve was separate and drew pictures of tiny bulbs at the end of individual nerve fibres that looked like little hands extending from one nerve cell to caress its neighbour (see Fig. 8.5).

Those who a few years earlier had used Golgi's new method to support their network theory of brain function were eventually forced to concede that Cajal was correct: each nerve cell in the brain was separate from every other nerve cell. In 1906 Golgi and Cajal shared the Nobel Prize for their discoveries.

With the recognition of the validity of 'the neuronal theory', some rapprochement between chemists who knew about mole-cules and physicists who knew about electricity might have occurred in brain science. This was not the case. The century-old commitment to brain electricity would not die easily; electricity remained the stuff of thought for many more decades.

One of the bright Cambridge graduates who visited Berlin in 1885 to learn about the cell from Rudolph Virchow was Charles

Sherrington (1857–1952). Sherrington returned to England and established first in Liverpool and later in Oxford a laboratory that was the centre of experimental neurology. He was the first to grasp the significance of the caressing paws that Cajal had found on nerve endings and gave them the name 'synapse', borrowing from the Greek word for 'clasp'.

Starting with a conviction that all nervous information must be transferred across the synapse, but not able to measure that transfer, Sherrington performed surgical experiments that demonstrated the importance of the synapse to brain function and was able to discern relationships between groups of neurons that depended upon synapses. Sherrington deduced that controlling information from thousands of individual nerve cells must be funnelled into a 'final common pathway'. He also described a 'reflex arc', which brought information into the nervous system and dumped it into the final common pathway, which in turn carried it out of the nervous system.

To those brain scientists who held to the network theory, synapses were disastrous 'circuit breakers'; it was difficult to see how electrical currents could scoot around inside the brain if circuits were not continuous. But more than that, the presence of synapses suggested that body juices could leak into these spaces. The uncertainty that synapses brought to the concept of a 'hard-

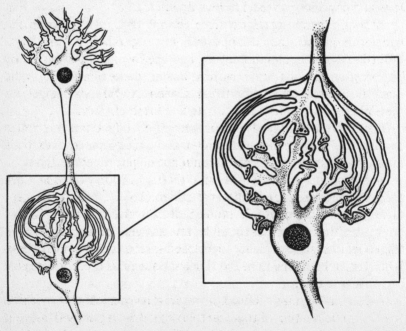

Fig. 8.5 Synapses: 'clasping paws' that connect nerves

wired' brain threatened the supremacy not only of Galvani's electricity, but also of the brain over the body.

Sherrington's laboratory became Mecca for brain scientists from all over the world, especially Americans. Those who visited saw experiments that were almost entirely geared to the eventual understanding of the circuitry of the brain. To Sherrington's Liverpool laboratory came Harvey Cushing, the father of modern neurosurgery, to join in experimental operations on apes. When he returned to Baltimore and began to perform neurosurgery, Cushing was quick to stimulate the cortex of a human with an electrical current much as he had done in Liverpool on apes.

The report of that operation (on 6 July 1908) seemed to confirm dramatically that the human brain was driven by the same stuff that made Galvani's frog legs twitch: electricity. Cushing did not do more with brain electricity; in that same year he switched his energies dramatically to the understanding of the endocrinology of the brain, especially the pituitary. But in the decades that followed, other neurosurgeons performed many different kinds of operations based on the premise that electricity was the stuff of thought, most of which were only copies of Sherrington's animal operations. The blessing that neurosurgeons gave to Sherrington's notions that the 'integration' of the nervous system depended upon its hard wires did much to ensure that other clinical disciplines, especially neurology and psychiatry, would follow along.

Although many of Sherrington's precepts were helpful to bedside diagnosis, they left physicians trying to help patients with brain disease without ammunition. In some cases it was worse. The Sherrington-like surgical modifications of the nervous system did more harm than good. For these reasons a still-existing schism developed between brain scientists and brain physicians.

Sherrington employed the techniques of reductionistic science to take the brain apart into smaller and smaller pieces; but once apart, like Humpty-Dumpty, it could not be put together again.

Many aspects of Dalton's atomic theory (1809), Schwann's cell theory (1839), Bernard's internal milieu (1856), Cajal's synapses (1895), and Sherrington's studies of neural integration (1906) suggested that molecules might be important to brain function, but the belief in brain electricity foreclosed serious study of that possibility for more than a century. The brain was an electrical organ, and that was that.

In 1924 in Germany, Otto Loewi found a chemical that modified the rhythmic beating of the heart; he called it 'vagus stuff' since it clearly came from the vagus nerve. When analysed by chemists, it was found to be acetylcholine. One of the young Jewish scientists working there, Wilhelm Feldberg, was forced to flee to England where he came to work for Sir Henry Dale. In his head he carried the specific information about acetylcholine measurements, and in 1934 he began to look for acetylcholine in the nerve endings that are attached to muscles. In twenty-six scientific papers Dale and Feldberg described the presence of acetylcholine in these nerve-muscle synapses, but in 1936 Feldberg was forced to leave the laboratory because of 'lack of support'. He went to Australia where almost immediately he received a letter saying that Dale planned to publish the chemical neurotransmission story without his name. Quickly and quietly Feldberg singlehandedly published a paper describing 'chemical neurotransmission'. Dale's subsequent paper omitted Feldberg's name but for more than one year Feldberg's obscure publication was the best source for the 'truth' about chemical neurotransmission. Dale and Loewi shared the Nobel Prize for chemical neurotransmission and shortly afterwards Feldberg returned to England.

Acetylcholine was the first chemical linked to the electrical signal that is measured on the surface of nerves, but in short order there were several others including noradrenaline, adrenaline, dopamine and serotonin. It appeared to Dale and his colleagues that these 'neurotransmitters' were produced by the nerve and carried to the synapse; on their release in the synaptic cleft, an electric signal passed from one nerve to another.

In this concept of synaptic transmission, held for forty years, it was assumed that one nerve contained one kind of neurotransmitter. Nerves were designated by the chemical signal that each contained: some nerves were adrenergic, some serotonergic and some dopaminergic, and so on (ergic = 'driven'). This concept became known as Dale's law, but we see in it a grudging kind of willingness on the part of brain electricians to let molecules into the brain. If they were present at all, it was only in the synaptic cleft, and then one nerve could only have one molecule. Now we know that Dale's law is in error. Many nerves contain many different kinds of neurotransmitters (see Fig 8.5).

The discovery of chemical neurotransmission did not dissuade brain scientists from their commitment to brain electricity. Dale's discovery only enhanced the scientific nobility of Galvani's brain electricity.

The advent of the electronmicroscope made it easy to peek in at the nerve fibres and see the little 'balls' of neurotransmitters that are stored there (see Fig. 8.6). Such pictures, first available in

1958, seemed to put the minds of the brain electricians at ease: neurotransmitters were positioned at a place where they could push 'sparks' from one nerve to the next.

As the creative genius of America's many clever electricians became more obvious, the centre of electrically based brain studies moved to this country. The forerunner of the television set, the cathode ray oscilloscope, was the invention that capped the brain electricians' efforts. Before the oscilloscope, scientists had been forced to employ the 'smoked drum', a mechanical device that recorded muscle movement as a scratch on a moving roll of soot-black paper. The oscilloscope provided electronic amplification of very weak signals and it, more than any other scientific tool, glued the brain to the bench of brain electricians. They could measure the tiniest sparks, even those in the synapse. As the cathode ray tube became central to both television and the computer, the notion that electricity was central to the brain's internal communications was buttressed. Most brain scientists believed that this provided convincing, irrefutable evidence that the brain was a biological computer.

By stimulating in one part of the nerve and recording in another, Herbert Gasser and Joseph Erlanger were able to confirm that electrical signals were carried along the nerve at different rates of speed. Using this technique, they found that the velocity of conduction of nerve fibres was dependent upon the diameter of the nerve; large nerve fibres carried impulses very rapidly and smaller nerves more slowly. For these recordings, Gasser and Erlanger shared the Nobel Prize.

One of the first tissues to be examined with the electronmicroscope was nerve, and to everyone's surprise the material that wrapped Gasser's nerve fibres was little more than a jelly-roll wrapping composed of Schwann cells.

As oscilloscopes were linked to computers, the similarities between the brain and the computer became clearer. The reverberating circuits of the computer were described as 'cybernetic currents' by Norbert Weiner in 1948, and many scientists proposed elegant theories designed to prove that brain electricity, flowing in never-ending circuits, was the stuff of thought. Today, many people still believe that cybernetic currents reverberate in the brain. Some of the observations that have come from neurosurgical operating theatres have done much to support this concept, but perhaps the greatest boost for the cybernetic theory of brain function was the electroencephalograph. Invented by Hans Berger in Germany in 1924, it is now commonly linked to the computer. To many who see them, the sparks emanating from this mechanical marriage of the computer to the brain validate the paradigm that the brain is an electrically driven computer.

Perhaps the best known brain operation that came to the bedside from the laboratories of the brain electricians is 'frontal lobotomy'. This operation is the natural outgrowth of a scientific belief in an electrically driven brain. The inventor of frontal lobotomy, Egas Moniz of Portugal, was given a Nobel Prize for it, yet it sprang from the behavioural changes in an experimental monkey called 'Becky'. The social and medical disaster of lobotomy can be traced directly to this one hastily done, wrongly interpreted neurosurgical experiment.

This operation has been discredited enough already; but if scientists say that the brain is composed of hard-wired, dry circuits like a wire-filled computer, then those doctors who care for patients with brain illnesses might be excused for cutting the circuits of the brain or for overstimulating the circuits – giving electroconvulsive therapy – for both are logical endpoints of that paradigm.

A far greater neurosurgical mismeme was created in this era. In 1911, Walter Dandy, a neurosurgeon in Baltimore, performed experiments that were just as bad as those on 'Becky'. Dandy

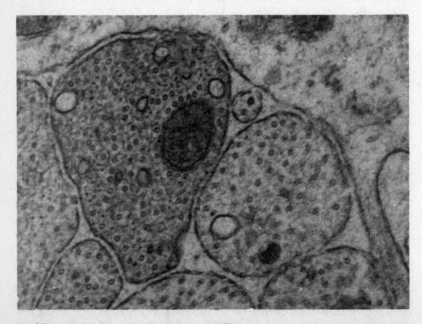

Fig. 8.6 An electronmicrograph of cut-across nerve fibres

postulated that brain water was formed solely as a 'hydraulic cushion' for the electrically driven brain. In doing this he gave the world a false *raison d'être* for the hollowness of the brain and allowed the best physiologists of the day to focus exclusively on the electrical circuits of the brain. It was Dandy's paradigm for brain water more than any other factor that allowed brain scientists to focus on the sparks rather than the juices of the brain. He also based much of his paradigm on an observation in a single experimental animal. Dandy's mistake was far more important than that of Egas Moniz.

Dandy's paradigm for brain water has provided a paradigm which at once keeps the brain 'dry' and gives brain scientists a false answer to the most important question in biology: 'Why is the brain hollow?'

Shoreline of Wonder

The brain became an electrical organ before any of the details were known about electricity itself, before the battery, dynamo and motor, and long before the electrically based devices of communications. After Galvani the brain became a testing ground for the best gadgets of electricians, who were not so much interested in the brain as in the demonstration of their newest and finest equipment. Their devices did demonstrate electrical currents emanating from the brain and from individual nerves. And as these same devices were employed in communications – telegraphs, telephones, radios, and much later television – both physicists and biologists jointly concluded that electrical signals were also responsible for communications in the brain.

Linking electricity to the brain gave electricity nobility. But the reverse also happened: brain biologists, able to link their subject of inquiry to the most exciting branch of science, slipped their research activities into the exciting mainstream of scientific inquiry. For most of this century, the study of brain electricity has been the darling endeavour of the research community. Whole buildings and entire divisions of academic institutions have been focused on the mysterious stuff that makes frog legs twitch; only a casual glance at Nobel awards, Royal Society rosters, or National Institute of Health grants can demonstrate how much our society has believed that some good would come from the effort to know more about the electrical currents in the brain.

These research efforts, however, have done very little for patient care. Physicians who have been left at the bedside without scientific partners, wondering why so much is known about the rat brain and so little about the human brain, will now have an alternative: they can look to endocrine-based laboratories in the knowledge that hormones drive the mind.

Julius Axelrod, the Nobel laureate who knows most about synaptic chemistry, wrote in September 1984: 'Ten years ago only three or four neurotransmitters had been recognized; now about fifty . . . have been identified. It now appears that the brain is a complex endocrine organ that releases a variety of hormone-like peptides.' That statement succinctly summarizes the dramatic revolution in brain biology that has occurred in the past decade; a two-century long scientific commitment to brain electricity has been replaced by an interest in brain hormones.

9

Confiteor: Neurosurgical Malfeasances

L et me tell you about my involvement in a tragedy. Elise had been the leading dancer in one of the world's best ballet companies. She had given the best hours of every day since childhood to the dance and had come to love her lithe, strong legs. Born slightly bow-legged, she had recognized early on in her career that this gave her tremendous leaping ability.

At the age of thirty, at the pinnacle of her success, disaster struck. Over a two-day period she developed total paralysis of both legs. Her doctors, the best in the world, diagnosed her condition as 'transverse myelitis' and listed the possible causes. Some had been optimistic at the beginning, but as the weeks wore on and there was no sign of recovery the truth was clear: she would never move her legs again.

In the years that followed, the numb sensation in her paralysed legs was replaced by a sensation of pain. Woefully, any stimulation of her legs, the lightest touch, the weight of the bedclothes, a breeze, would cause a crescendo of pain so severe that she cried out in anguish.

The doctors, again the best in the world, called this 'anesthesia dolorosa', a condition in which the anesthetic parts of her body were painful.

Her pain separated her from her supportive friends and bound her more and more to her doctors. Soon an appetite for food was replaced by an appetite for narcotics. Then a love of narcotics became the driving force in her life but, even in doses strong enough to cause sleep, her pain never relented.

Fifteen years after the illness began I was asked to see her by a physician who was more conservative than most. He suggested that I surgically remove her spinal cord. He argued that it was no good to her, and that some kind of crooked regeneration had occurred within it that allowed touch sensation, or any sensation, to be interpreted by her brain as 'pain'. As I had done more than my share of spinal surgery, he selected me to perform this heroic, desperate procedure. The operation was intended to rid Elise of the unbearable, untreatable pain in her legs. She would trade her persistent pain for persistent numbness.

At operation, I made a lengthy midline incision in the upper back, removed the bones that formed the roof of the spinal canal and removed all the spinal cord below the level of the myelitis. The cord was abnormally small and abnormally coloured – certainly dead – and as I closed the wound I was confident that cord removal was the correct choice.

When Elise awoke from the operation her hopes, her husband's hopes, her personal physician's hopes, her nurse's hopes and my hopes were crushed. Her pain continued as before, not changed one bit by my heroic removal of her spinal cord.

The operation on Elise stemmed from the studies of anatomists who had located the 'pain pathway'. Knowing that many millions of nerves connected the body to the brain, they separated out the bundles that carried pain messages. They had reduced the problem of pain to a one-way signal, and my failed operation was based on that simplistic reduction of a very complex problem. It was my faith in that paradigm that led me to perform every kind of nerve-cutting operation for pain that has been devised.

Most of my operations for pain have failed in one way or another, and I have lost confidence in my ability to relieve pain by surgical procedures. Only in patients with facial pain – 'trigeminal neuralgia' – can I confidently predict a successful outcome of a destructive operation.

Now, fifteen years after my operation on Elise, it is obvious to me and to most brain scientists that the brain is a gland. Pain is not something that can be effectively treated by dividing electrical circuits in the brain. Now we know that brain hormones modulate virtually every aspect of pain; the brain makes its own opiate-like hormones, enkephalin and endorphin, and has its own opiate receptors. It is the interaction of these hormones and receptors that underlie pain tolerance, pain intolerance and addiction to pain-relieving drugs. But many other brain hormones besides enkephalin and endorphin are involved in pain modulation; somatostatin, cholecystokinen, vasopressin, substance P, vasoactive intestinal peptide and neurotensin all may be involved. Each hormone appears to be effective by virtue of hormone and hormone receptor interaction in much the same way as the opiate and opiate receptor relationship. Each of the new brain peptides that are involved in pain modulation seems to interact with the others in patterns that are complex, but increasingly it is apparent that the electrical signals that are involved in pain are akin to the sparks that are produced by a fire. Hormones in the brain govern the fires that produce these sparks.

The reductionism of the paradigm that the brain is an electrically driven computer gave a narrowly focused, at best, half-true, starting premise to all brain doctors. Knowing now of the holistic relationships that are involved between brain and body hormones makes our electrically based reductionistic therapies appear not only wrong but also dumb.

My disastrous experience with Elise came shortly after the 'gate-control' theory of pain had been described in 1965. This revolutionary concept was advanced in that year by Patrick Wall and Ronald Melzack, and it provided a rational explanation for the failure of nerve-cutting operations to relieve pain.

The gate-control theory proposed that nature has set in place two very different systems that carry pain messages to the brain. Although they work together, nature has given us one system that protects us from outer injury during attack, and another that protects us from inner injury, from hurting ourselves.

This paradigm for pain modulation is named 'gate control' because one of these systems closes gates after the first news of pain reaches the brain. The other opens gates after the first pain message is sent to the brain.

Nature has given humans a wonderful mechanism that closes the gates through which pain signals must pass on their way to the brain. This mechanism is ordained to protect us from outside injury. If someone is attacked and physically wounded, for example, the initial pain serves as an alerting mechanism. But quickly the gates close, and the individual is able to carry on in defence without thinking of the painful wound. This mechanism is set in place for one purpose: to protect the body from external attack. The mechanism must be quick and is carried to the brain along the largest nerves, which carry the fastest signals (see Fig. 8.3). The mechanism must be sensitive and is carried by nerves that have the most sensitive hair triggers. But once the quick, sensitive mechanism is activated, it closes the gates through which it passed.

This gate-closing mechanism is seen commonly by those of us who man emergency rooms for accident victims or battalion hospitals for soldiers. There it is often observed that very severely injured people do not complain of pain. You have probably experienced the protection of the gate-closing mechanism: when the human thumb touches a hot stove or is slammed by a misdirected hammer, the initial pain pulls the hand back by reflex action. Then for a few minutes the gates are closed and the intensity of the pain is greatly diminished. It is later in the day, or in the night, when the gates are open again that the full intensity of the pain is appreciated by the brain. This is a common experience which did not rouse much scientific curiosity until 1965.

Nature carries pain originating inside the body by a different mechanism. This one is slow; there is no need for quick reflex movement, and it can be carried along thin, delicate nerve fibres at a slow rate. It is not very sensitive, and the stimuli that activate it must push against firm triggers, not hair triggers. But once these signals are carried by this mechanism to the brain, they open the gates through which they passed. Once open, these gates will allow even mild stimuli, those that ordinarily would not be at all bothersome, to reach the brain and to be interpreted as pain.

Together these two systems provide a beautifully balanced defence: the gate-closing mechanism protects against external injury, and the gate-opening mechanism protects against internal injury – against disease.

Most of the chronic pains that come to humans are carried by the slow-conducting mechanisms that open gates. Arthritis, disc disease, stomach cramps and angina are typical examples of internal causes of pain. Nature wants such patients to rest, not necessarily to take to their bed, but at least, to take it easy, confident that rest will cure the pain-causing problems. As patients with such pain know well, once the gate-opening mechanism is activated, all kinds of ordinary and non-noxious stimuli are perceived by the brain as painful.

The hinges of these gates can be controlled by the brain. Some signals flow out from the brain to set the tension of the gates. The gates can be adjusted by the brain to stay in the closed position. The Indian fakir lying on a bed of nails has developed such control over his pain-modulating gates that he can close them at will and limit the number of pain signals that reach his brain. The harried housewife who is insecure, lonely and depressed, on the other hand, cannot muster the brain energy to put any pressure on the brain side of the gates that control pain. Without that force coming from the brain, her gates stay open. Any sensation can pass through the gates and on to the brain. Backache, neckache and headache are the natural consequences of this situation. The pains are not imagined, they are real, but they result from a change in the threshold of gate opening and closing, not from any real disease in the back, the neck or the head.

The gate-control theory makes good sense, and for less than five years gate control appeared to be the best paradigm for understanding and treating pain. Like many others in my profession, I welcomed it, for it gave me a reason to slow down on nerve-cutting operations and a rational explanation for my failures.

During the time that the details of the gate-control paradigm were being worked out, America was racing to the moon. A crucial aspect of the moonshot programme was the ability of our scientists to broadcast radio signals to distant satellites.

The gate-control paradigm depended upon two kinds of nerves: one had a firm trigger and the other a hair trigger. The nerves that closed gates required only a one millivolt stimulus; the nerves that opened gates required a stimulus ten times as strong: ten millivolts.

This difference in threshold made electrical counterstimulation possible; brain scientists knew that a low-powered stimulus would close gates and not be interpreted as pain. To moonshot scientists, broadcasting radio signals into the brain or spinal cord was far less difficult than broadcasting to and from distant satellites. Knowing that there was a ten-fold difference between the gate-closing stimulus and the gate-opening stimulus made their task easier.

Two devices came off the NASA shelves and on to the shelves of neurosurgeons which allowed electrical counterstimulation to be used in patient care. Both depended upon the very sensitive nerves that closed gates; both were designed with the hope that a scarcely detectable 'buzz' could replace high-intensity pain.

The simplest of these is the 'transcutaneous electrical nerve stimulator', or TENS, a battery-operated device that delivers an electrical signal to a nerve located just below the skin. The TENS has the sophisticated space-age miniaturization that allows the patient to twist the dials of the device to a frequency and strength that closes gates and reduces the brain's perception of pain.

A more complicated device is the 'dorsal column stimulator', an ingenious radio receiver/transmitter that can be implanted permanently beneath the skin. The signal of this internal broadcasting station is carried along wires beneath the skin to platinum electrodes that are placed on the surface of the spinal cord. The radio does not have its own power supply; it is turned on by a battery-operated 'wand' or external coil that is held over the skin just above the receiver/transmitter. Activating the battery pack turns on the radio station, which sends its signals to the dorsal columns of the spinal cord.

It seemed then, in 1970, that the gate-control theory was a happy marriage of mankind's two greatest intellectual frontiers, the mind and space.

For the next few years, thousands of dorsal column stimulators were implanted with results that were far less impressive than the gate-control paradigm would have predicted. This electrically based paradigm for brain function looked wonderful in the laboratory but, at the bedside, didn't work well at all. The operation is seldom done today.

The TENS device, because it is innocuous, is still used widely, and many claim that it is the Western equivalent of acupuncture. In my experience it is helpful in about one third of patients, but placebo medications may match that level of effectiveness.

Dorsal column stimulation and percutaneous stimulation have been therapeutic failures, certainly not the panacea for pain. Despite those failures, the gate-control theory of pain modulation is valid. It is certainly the most useful paradigm that a patient in pain can know, for it encourages the use of the gate-closing ability that lies dormant in the brain.

My surgical failures – first in attempts to break the circuits of the brain and second in attempts to stimulate the circuits of the brain – are recounted to underscore the failure of the paradigm that the brain is an electrically driven computer. However easily electrical potentials can be measured on the surface of individual nerves or on the surface of the brain, when this paradigm is taken to the bedside it is not very helpful. Yet from the story of gate-control comes one of the best surprises in the history of the mind: as scientists sought an explanation for this phenomenon – for the pain tolerance of the Indian fakir and the pain-intolerance of the harried housewife – they came to realize that the brain is a gland. Hormones, not electricity, determine all brain/body and brain/behavioural relationships.

Shoreline of Wonder

If you have accepted the double-think of modern medicine and science – 'Molecules shape the body, but electricity shapes the mind' – you have unwittingly limited what your brain can do.

Why?

Electricity, of any kind, is something that you fear; you cannot control it. The terror of its shock, the sight of its spark, and the lightning bolt are long-lasting lessons that this stuff is not easily managed. Its control can only come by reduction: transformers reduce its power, insulators reduce its threat, switches reduce its pathways. You give away that controlling reduction to someone else – to the power companies that reduce current, to the manufacturers who insulate wires and to the electricians who direct the currents through your home.

If you believe that electricity is the stuff of thought, you will treat your brain like anything else electrical; when things go wrong inside it, you will seek an outside expert – a doctor – much as you seek an outside expert for your radio, telephone, or television set.

Your doctor, motivated in part by the honest belief that you are unable to cope, too often will assume it is a therapeutic duty to reduce brain power with sleeping pills, insulate brain activity with tranquillizers, or direct the brain's patterns of thought by analysis.

But more important, accepting the notion that the brain is an electrically driven computer makes it impossible for you to consider the therapeutic option of adding something to the brain that could make it work more efficiently and effectively; reduction is your only option. You are then trapped by the silent snares of Western science: breaking things into smaller and smaller bits – reductionism – is espoused, for smaller things are more easily controlled; joining things together into a larger whole – holism – is eschewed, for control becomes more difficult.

The double-think that grows from scientific reductionism is as perilous to our society as a whole as it is to you as an individual. I can write about the pros and cons of Western reductionism as Conrad wrote about whaling: from personal experience. For much of my life I have been both a bedside doctor and a laboratory researcher. In both of these activities, reductionism – specialization – has been my driving mind mechanism.

Yet in the past decade laboratory studies of the brain have been given a new preamble: hormones moving from the brain to the body and from the body to the brain modulate every aspect of brain/behaviour relationships and brain/body relationships. In accepting this preamble, brain scientists have suddenly come to espouse holism and are trying to put together the bits and pieces of the brain that have been broken apart by their reductionistic forefathers.

The new paradigm views the brain as a complex whole, an organ that does not stand apart from the rest of the body, run by different stuff, but shares the same internal milieu as other organs. At first glance the new holistic understanding of brain hormones seems mind-boggling, too complex to either understand or to be useful in designing better forms of therapy. But we now have no choice: we must acknowledge the unity of the brain and the body, admit that brain hormones are really body hormones and recognize that hormonal therapies aimed at making the brain whole again must replace reductionistic therapies aimed at bridling its electrical currents.

10

The Giants of the Brain Gland

To academic surgeons, the names John Hunter, William Halsted, and Harvey Cushing have a ring that matches those of Socrates, Plato and Aristotle. As the three ancient Greeks set in place guidelines for Western thought, the three surgeons established the principles that have guided Western surgery. Remarkably, each of these surgeons contributed significantly to the understanding of endocrinology, and their individual paradigms came together as the foundation stones for a new science, neuroendocrinology.

Medical historians rank John Hunter (1728–93) as medicine's greatest creative genius; he is most remarkable because he never received any formal education. The principles of infectious disease, immunization, bone growth, inflammation and lymphatic flow are a few of his discoveries. Many count him as the father of endocrinology, because he understood so clearly that endocrine organs influence behaviour and body function. He was the first to transplant glands, and those experiments are still on display in his museum in London.

Noting the changed behaviour in a hen that had received the transplanted testicles of a cock, Hunter said: 'The testicles are the cause of changed inclinations, yet they do not direct these inclinations. The inclinations become an operation of the mind after the mind is once stimulated by the testicle.'

Hunter did many remarkable things. Most notable, some might say, was his self-inoculation with the germs of syphillis to ascertain that it was an infectious disease. But in the years that follow historians may recognize that his discovery of the hormonal control of the mind was his greatest contribution.

Fred Mettler, an eminent medical historian, has accumulated evidence to demonstrate that Hunter's lack of education stems from severe dyslexia. It was this handicap that forced him to observe things for himself and to store his observations in bottles, rather than in words. Two decades after Hunter died, his papers were burned by a close associate. This earned Hunter's friend the wrath of academic Britain, but Mettler believes it was a noble gesture performed to protect Hunter's academic reputation: it appears the papers were written in someone else's hand. Hunter may have been nearly illiterate.

William Halsted (1856–1922) is regarded as the father of American surgery. He was one of the four people who established America's premier academic medical school, Johns Hopkins, and the inventor of many operations, a new operative technique, rubber gloves, endocrine surgery and the strategy of residency education for young surgeons. Before the science of endocrinology was invented, Halsted had worked out the basic principles of the surgical transplantation of glands; in doing that he was retracing steps taken by John Hunter a century before.

Halsted became addicted to opiates while at Bellevue Hospital where, soon after the invention of hollow needles and syringes, he used himself as a guinea pig to work out the details of local anaesthesia. Although he spent time in treatment, he never escaped his habit. He was recruited to Baltimore where he remained productive both in the laboratory and in the operating room.

Harvey Cushing (1869–1939) is regarded as the father of neurosurgery. He had attended Yale College and Harvard Medical School but sought out Halsted for his surgical training. Cushing singlehandedly developed the surgical specialty of neurosurgery, while maintaining an active role in the laboratory. His legendary experiments in the first decade of this century established that the pituitary gland controlled the function of other endocrine glands.

Cushing was in many ways very much like Hunter; both were interested in dwarfs and giants, both devised new methods of controlling bleeding, both were interested in new and better ways of treating infected wounds, both were military surgeons, both were collectors – Hunter of biological specimens and Cushing of books – and both affixed their names to medical diseases: the penile ulcer of syphillis was called the 'Hunterian chancre' and excessive adrenal gland activity was called 'Cushing's disease'.

In another way Hunter and Cushing were very different: while Hunter did not leave a written legacy, Cushing was a prolific, gifted writer: his two-volume work on the life of William Osler won him the Pulitzer Prize.

Most remarkably, Hunter and Cushing collaborated in the evaluation of a patient, Charles O'Brien, although they were separated by more than a century.

Hunter's energies led him to collect 10,000 biological specimens, and to that collection came the wired-together skeleton of
Charles O'Brien, a carnival giant more than eight feet tall.
Referred to as the 'Irish Giant', O'Brien died when he was twenty-
two, and newspapers reported that he was buried at sea, but two
years later a human skeleton that was eight feet tall appeared in
Hunter's collection. It is still in London in the Hunterian Museum.

In 1910, shortly after Cushing had demonstrated that the pituitary was responsible for growth, he visited the John Hunter
Museum and asked the curator, Sir Arthur Keith (who discovered
the nerves of the heart), to saw open the giant's skull to see if a
pituitary tumour had been the cause of his great growth. Keith
obliged, and they found the bone erosion that is typical of a pituitary tumour. This was very important to Cushing's research,
because it confirmed that the pituitary secreted a substance, now
called growth hormone, which caused the body to grow. In
O'Brien's case, the pituitary tumour that had caused the erosion of
the base of his skull had secreted excessive amounts of growth
hormone.

These three surgeons – John Hunter, William Halsted, and
Harvey Cushing – all fit Koestler's description of genius:

Most geniuses responsible for the major mutations in the history of
thought seem to have certain features in common; on the one hand scep-
ticism, often carried to the point of iconoclasm, in their attitude towards
traditional ideas, axioms, and dogmas, towards everything that is taken
for granted; on the other hand, an open-mindedness that verges on naive
credulity towards new concepts which seem to hold out some promise to
their instinctive gropings. Out of this combination results that crucial
capacity of perceiving a familiar object, situation, problem, or collection of
data, in a sudden new light or new context; of seeing a branch not as part
of a tree, but as a potential weapon or tool; of associating the fall of an
apple not with its ripeness, but with the motion of the moon. The
discoverer perceives relational patterns of functional analogies where
nobody saw them before.

The new 'relational patterns' that Hunter saw in physiology,
Halsted saw in wound healing, and Cushing saw in the pituitary
were formed in the pattern-recognizing right brain of each.

In the last few decades there have been few, if any, surgeons
who have contributed to the fundamental understanding of the
endocrine system. Surgeons must be holists, and as scientific
endeavours have become increasingly reductionistic, they have
become less involved in laboratory studies. Yet the scientists who

picked up the torch passed from Hunter to Halsted to Cushing have
been a breed apart; they, too, have eschewed the scientific reductionism of their colleagues in favour of holistic attempts to bring
the endocrine system and the nervous system together. These
men were also remarkable for their ability to put together new
'relational patterns' from the bits and pieces other biologists had
taken apart.

Their holistic endeavours have been of two kinds. The first
focused on the control that the brain exerts over the glands of the
body; these resulted in a branch of science that is called 'neuroendocrinology' and began in 1932. The second is concerned with
the effects that the glands have upon the brain; this science is
called 'endocrine neurology' and began less than a decade ago.

The man who conceived of the notion that the brain could convey
its commands by hormones was Joe Hinsey, and the man who
verified that this happened was Geoffrey Harris.

Hinsey might be regarded as the 'architect' of the first bridge
from the brain to the endocrine system. A superb physiologist and
anatomist, he made the observation in 1932, against established
dogma, that the anterior pituitary gland contained no nerves. As an
Iowa-born farmboy, Hinsey was well aware that after sexual coitus
many female animals release eggs from their ovaries. In the
experimental laboratory he was able to verify that the insertion of
a glass rod into the vagina of females of these species would do the
same thing. To prove that the pituitary was important to reflex
ovulation, he removed the pituitary in some animals and found that
post-coital ovulation did not occur; the pituitary was the essential
link. But how could the information get from the stimulated vagina
to the pituitary if there were no nerves in the pituitary?

In other unrelated studies Hinsey had observed that 'juices'
were released from nerve endings into the surrounding tissue. He
postulated that something similar must be happening in the pituitary. Some tissue juice, a molecular messenger, must carry the
brain's information to the pituitary. Hinsey's very simple experiments with reflex ovulation were the first steps in the realization
that the brain is a gland.

One mind that Hinsey's meme infiltrated was that of George
Wislocki, the anatomist at Harvard who demonstrated the route
that Hinsey's tissue juices could take to the nerveless pituitary.
Wislocki brought together Hinsey's observations and those of
Gregory Popa, an anatomist from Bucharest. In 1930 Popa was
briefly in England and called attention to the similarities between

the blood vessels at the base of the brain and those in the abdomen.

For centuries it had been known that a special circulation in the abdomen carried blood from 'portal to portal'. At one port, the gut, food was added to the blood and at the next port, the liver, this food was unloaded. These vessels became known as the 'portal system' but are merely veins that carry blood from one capillary bed to a second capillary bed without help from the arterial circulation.

Popa recognized that the blood vessels he had discovered at the base of the brain were 'portal vessels'; one capillary bed was in the brain and the other capillary bed was in the pituitary. He postulated that they carried blood from the pituitary to the brain. Had he known of Hinsey's deduction that molecular information was carried from the brain to the pituitary, doubtless he would have postulated that these blood vessels carried blood in the opposite direction: from the brain to the pituitary.

In 1935 Wislocki confirmed that Popa's portal vessels existed, but he claimed that they carried blood in the opposite direction, from the brain to the pituitary. With that suggestion Wislocki laid the anatomical cornerstone for neuroendocrinology.

Wislocki regarded the capillaries at the base of the brain as a 'vascular switchyard', much like the train tracks in a railroad yard, which could direct some brain molecules to the body and others to the anterior pituitary. Brain scientists, knowing about this, designed concepts that split the hormonal functions of the brain in two: one part, they contended, would make molecules destined for the body and the other part would make molecules destined for the pituitary (see Fig. 10.1).

Wislocki's vascular switchyard became the conceptual equivalent of a signal converter, a transducer, which converted electrical signals into molecular signals. That view is taught in most basic books of science today even though it is not wholly correct.

Inherent in Wislocki's paradigm for brain-pituitary relationships was an insistence that all the blood in the switchyard was flowing 'south' towards the pituitary. That view separated an 'electrical' brain from a 'hormonal' endocrine system and set people thinking that electricity was flowing 'south' to the pituitary and that hormones, in turn, were flowing 'south' to the body.

After my neurosurgical training, I spent several years in anatomical laboratories looking closely at the pituitary. Many of my studies were focused on the blood vessels that connect the brain to the pituitary. As certainly as Wislocki's studies suggested

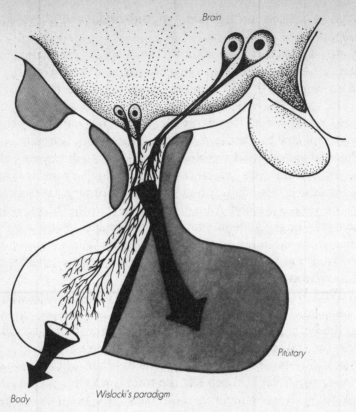

Fig. 10.1 The portal veins of the pituitary, showing the vascular channels that blood can take from the brain to the pituitary

to him that the brain's secretions were carried 'south', my studies suggested that some hormones might be carried from the vascular switchyard 'north' to the brain.

My studies demonstrated five different routes by which hormones could be carried from the pituitary directly to the brain. I cannot accept Wislocki's notion that a vascular switchyard separates an electrically driven brain from a hormonally driven endocrine system. The switchyard that Wislocki described unites two glands: the brain and the pituitary.

There is evidence that brain hormones do pass along the pathway that Hinsey and Wislocki found; it was the biochemists who followed these anatomists down the pathway that led to the major advances in neuroendocrinology.

One of these biochemists was Vincent du Vigneaud (1901–80), head of biochemistry at Cornell Medical School, who was awarded the Nobel Prize for the synthesis of the first peptide hormone, 'vasopressin'. This hormone is made in the brain and is carried by nerves into the switchyard that Wislocki described. It is stored in nerve endings there until the command comes from the brain for its release.

Vasopressin is a 'protein', and as such, one of the basic building blocks of the body. The term 'protein' is derived from the word 'protus', meaning 'first stuff'. The tiny granules that form these blocks, the molecules, are called 'amino-acids' and these are often joined together like beads of a necklace. There are only twenty 'essential' amino-acids, and they serve in the formation of proteins much like letters of an alphabet are employed to form words. Du Vigneaud was the first to untangle a protein necklace and put it back together again. He did this for vasopressin and its sister molecule oxytocin in 1954, and since then hundreds of other proteins have been untangled by scientists and produced synthetically.

In 1967 I was able to visualize in humans little 'balls' of vasopressin moving down the nerves projecting into Wislocki's switchyard (see Fig. 10.2). These granules are formed by the brain and conveyed in the nerve fibre, the axon, for nearly an inch. Sometimes these granules bunch up in a nerve fibre that looks like it is constipated; that is, material that one would assume to be moving 'down' towards the pituitary is held up for some unknown reason.

These constipated nerve fibres were seen by Cushing, using an optical microscope. He called them 'Herring bodies' and thought that they moved 'up' towards the brain not 'down' towards the pituitary. Cushing first said that in 1909 and maintained that view until he died in 1939; he believed this so fervently that in 1930 he ground up the pituitary gland and placed it in the ventricles of humans to see what would happen. Long before I suggested that pituitary secretions

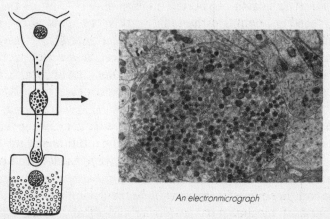

An electronmicrograph

Fig. 10.2 For forty years scientists thought that a 'vascular switchyard' in the pituitary stalk delivered some brain hormones to the anterior pituitary and other brain hormones to the body as shown

might be carried towards the brain, Cushing was doing experiments to test that possibility.

I believe that such injections offer great hope to those with many kinds of brain illness. But for many reasons, many of them legal, Cushing's experiments have never been repeated.

Two superbly creative anatomists, Ernst and Berta Scharrer, looked very carefully at the granules that were being transported down nerves. They concluded that this was a common occurrence not only in the pituitary but in virtually every nerve. They demonstrated, in insects, similar granules travelling from the brain to the heart to control the way the heart beats. They described three kinds of neuroendocrine relationships, each dependent on axonal transport of brain hormones. The Scharrers pointed all their arrows from the brain to the body but, as we will see later, hormones move both into the brain and out of it by nerve transport.

Without doubt the greatest contributor to the science of neuroendocrinology was Geoffrey Harris (1906–71) who, in his last years, was the head of anatomy at Oxford. Harris got his start in science by looking at the blood vessels that unite the brain and the pituitary; by chance he was at Cambridge when Popa was there writing about the pituitary portal vessels. Although much of Harris's life was spent on the trail outlined by Hinsey that led 'south' from the brain, he never lost his respect for Popa who proposed the opposite.

Harris was the first to prove that electrical signals were converted into molecular messages as Hinsey had suggested. Decades before miniaturized electronic gadgets, Harris implanted wires into the brains of rabbits, maintaining a 'coil' of the wire attached to the scalp. He then placed this strangely wired rabbit into the centre of a giant electrical induction coil. By passing a current through the outer coil, he generated an electric current in the wired rabbit. That current passed through the brain and, as you might predict, out popped an egg from the ovary.

Harris chased after the brain molecules that were released by electrical stimulation, knowing that this code would uncover the manner in which the brain controlled the pituitary. One of his students, however, Roger Guillemin, discovered that code first. To do that Guillemin had to harvest 5,000,000 tiny brain fragments from slaughterhouse sheep and reduce the accumulated fragments to a single milligram of material. By his reckoning the material that he recovered was more expensive, ounce for ounce, than the rocks that were returned from the moon.

Harris's work established that brain signals are converted into molecular messages that are carried by blood vessels to the pituitary. Tiny amounts of these molecules, probably the most powerful biological substances people have found, cause a 'cascade of amplification' that races from the brain to the pituitary and then to the whole body. At each step of this amplification process the signals are louder, last longer and influence more organs. His untangling of this complicated process resulted in a book, *The Neural Control of the Pituitary* and the fundamental paradigm of neuroendocrinology described in Fig. 10.3.

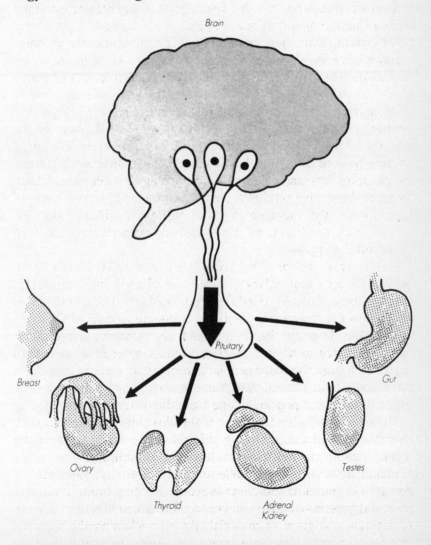

Fig. 10.3 Neuroendocrinology: brain hormones are released by nerves into the 'funnel' that drains into the anterior pituitary, which in turn releases hormones to more glands

During my years of neurosurgical education with Bronson Ray in New York, many hours were spent in the operating room focused on the human pituitary gland. It became obvious to us that many descriptions of the anatomy in this region were either incomplete or wrong. Encouraged by Bronson, I spent many years studying the pituitary. These studies confirmed what I had seen in the operating room: there were very few veins that drained the pituitary. It looked like the pituitary should explode. It was very easy to trace the pathway that blood took into it but very difficult to find veins that could carry blood out of it. Looking back at the drawings of Wislocki convinced me that he had not seen anterior pituitary veins either.

My anatomical observations have been deliberately interspersed between the discoveries of the giants of neuroendocrinology – Hunter, Halsted, Cushing, Hinsey, Wislocki, du Vigneaud, Scharrer, and Harris. My anatomical studies showed clear arrows pointing from the pituitary 'north' to the brain and set the stage for the accomplishments of later scientists, who in the past decade established that the same hormonal codes that flow from the brain to the glands of the body also flow in the reverse direction: from the glands to the brain. That information convinced scientists that hormones, not electricity, are the stuff of thought.

Shoreline of Wonder

It is the human mind, not the human body, which has shaped our civilization. The double-think of modern science, the view that 'molecules shape the body, but electricity shapes the mind', is lamentable. Is it possible that Western society has been built on a foundation of double-think? Has scientific reductionism sprung from the belief that human thoughts are electrical? Was 'reason' given the brittle qualities of a robot, and then pushed down a path which became increasingly mechanical, disjointed and competitive? Is the nuclear winter many anticipate the predictable consequence of the spiritual ice age that came from the notion that the brain is driven by fragmented, isolated electrons like a computer? Will the new view of the stuff of thought, which recognizes the importance of hormones, push the mind down a different path?

Noting that many of the giants who have shaped philosophy were also physicians, it may be that the principles of neuroendocrinology will have a greater impact on the shape of civilization than upon science itself. Thomas Kuhn notes that scientists often become concerned with philosophical matters during a scientific revolution, writing:

During a scientific revolution ... scientists take a different attitude toward existing paradigms, and the nature of their research changes accordingly. The proliferation of competing articulations, the willingness to try anything, the expression of explicit discontent, the recourse to philosophy and to debate over fundamentals – all these are the symptoms of a transition from normal to extraordinary research.

At present the world of brain science is in the middle of such a revolution. Scientists now regard the brain as a hormonally driven gland, not an electrically driven computer. Holism replaces reductionism in a new paradigm that gives human thoughts qualities that are warm, soft, wet, colourful, qualitative, timeless, communal and united.

In espousing the holism that is essential to neuroendocrinology, the pathfinders – John Hunter, William Halsted and Harvey Cushing – may have shown us not only a better way to think about thinking but also a better way to live.

11

The Year the Brain becomes a Gland

*T*he discoveries of Hinsey and Harris began the science of neuroendocrinology and gave the first clue that the stuff of thought might be something other than Galvani's brain electricity. This was the first suggestion that there might be another different, but equally defensible, view of the brain.

The search to understand the importance of brain hormones has produced a new branch of science, endocrine neurology, which acknowledges that hormones made in the body may influence the brain. The new paradigms that led to this changed way of thinking about the mechanics of the mind are shown in Fig. 11.1

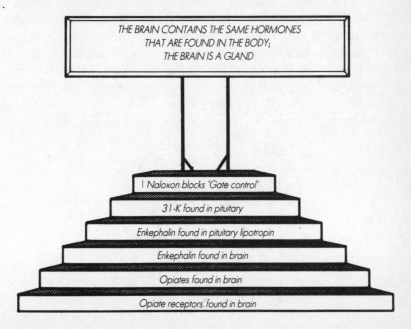

Fig. 11.1 The major steps taken by scientists as they came to know that the brain has all the qualities of a gland

Opium, the drug that separates the mind from the body, brought about this revolutionary holistic view of the brain and the body.

An accident of nature placed opium both in the brain and in the sap that flows from the seed pod of the poppy flower. Those who have tasted opium say that the pleasure it brings exceeds that of love, wine, food or any other drug. A very similar kind of bonding developed between opium and brain scientists. They found opium in the brain in 1975 and, like junkies, became hooked; brain opium became central to their dreams, and the search for it was filled with the frenzy of an addict in need of a fix. The scientific dalliance with this drug gave a new vision of the brain that reshaped all previous thoughts about thinking.

Because of its strong addictive powers, opium was banned in the United States despite pharmaceutical companies, doctors and patients recognizing that opium was the drug of choice for pain. Knowing this, pharmacologists began to make new synthetic drugs that would mimic the effect of opium but have less of its addictive qualities, and many of the tricks that were developed in the process became the wedges that split open the brain to reveal a cornucopia of brain hormones.

Thirty years ago, clever chemists constructed a synthetic molecule, naloxone, that had a structure similar to opium. But naloxone had no pain relieving ability; indeed, if an animal were given a naloxone injection, a later injection of opium had no effect. Quickly it was realized that naloxone was working like a dummy key; it would fit into a lock that was designed for opium but not open it. If it were stuck in the lock, the opium molecule could not work. These 'locks' are called 'receptors' by biologists and in this instance 'opiate receptors'. Naloxone was one of the first synthetic drugs that functioned as a 'receptor blocker' (see Fig. 11.2).

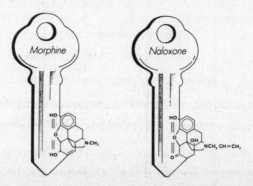

Fig. 11.2 The structure of the opiate drug morphine compared to the structure of naloxone, the opiate blocker

In Palo Alto in 1973, a pharmacologist, Avram Goldstein, demonstrated the presence of the opiate receptors in the brains of animals. Brains were homogenized in a machine very similar to a kitchen vegetable blender. This mush was placed in a funnel-shaped filter and different drugs poured through it. Generally, all the drugs came through the mush, but if there were receptors in the brain that would bind the drug, the drug would remain in the tissue in the funnel. By attaching a radioactive isotype to the drug and then measuring the radioactivity in the fluid that had been poured through the tissue, the presence or absence of specific receptors could be determined. Goldstein found opium receptors in the brain by this method. If opiate-like drugs such as heroin were poured through the brain, they were bound. To confirm this, naloxone was poured through the brain first; like a 'dummy key', it stuck into the 'lock' of the opium receptor. Then drugs such as heroin could be poured through the brain without binding. This was evidence that the brain contained opiate receptors.

Goldstein employed this technique to find that most opiate-like drugs were bound by brain tissue. In the next few months, opiate receptors were localized in very specific parts of the brain by scientists working in Baltimore, New York and Sweden.

Almost in unison scientists asked, 'Is the brain a gland? Does it have its own set of opium receptors and its own opium? Is it organized in such a way that it can treat itself? Can it give itself its own 'high' by the release of its internal opium?' By 1975 it was verified that the brain produced its own opiate-like hormones.

The vas deferens is the tiny tube that carries sperm from the testes to the urethra in males. For reasons that are clear to no one, the vas deferens has opiate receptors; when these are bound to an opiate, the vas deferens will contract vigorously.

To see if a new drug behaves like an opiate, a small strip of vas deferens from a mouse or a guinea pig is placed in a bath of fluid with one end attached to the bottom of the bath and the other end to a gauge at the top of the bath. The gauge records the muscle's movement. If an opiate is placed in the surrounding fluid, the vas deferens will contract rhythmically.

If a new drug causes the vas deferens to contract, it is probably an opiate. To make this relationship more substantial, naloxone can be added to the fluid; if naloxone prevents the contractions, the new drug is bound by opiate receptors in the vas deferens. To the drug company performing these experiments, this suggests that the new drug would also bind to the brain's opiate receptors and, if so, could be useful in the treatment of pain.

The vas deferens test for opiate-like action has been part of the developmental process for nearly all the drug industry's new 'pain-killers'. Coupled to today's modern automated machines, this test can screen many thousands of drugs in a short time.

Armed with the information that opiate receptors were in the brain and stimulated by the hunch that an opiate-like substance might also be present in the brain, biochemists began to search for 'brain opiates'. The search began in much the same way as the search for opiate receptors. The brain was placed in a kitchen blender and reduced to a liquid slurry.

To search for brain opiates, the many different molecules present in the slurry can be placed in a special kind of track – a 'column' – and forced to 'race' through it. If the column is long enough, 'pure populations' of molecules will pass out of the end of the column, separated one from the other by their 'racing speed'.

It was this technique that was employed by John Hughes and Hans Kosterlitz in Aberdeen, Scotland, to conduct the winning search for brain opiates. As the molecules came racing out of the end of the column, each was placed in a bath containing the device that measured contractions of the vas deferens. Pig brains were used and, in a most important scientific report, in 1975, Hughes and Kosterlitz described opiate-like activity in one of the populations of brain molecules.

Once this molecule was found and isolated in the brain, there was a race to understand the chemical structure of this molecule; scientists were keenly aware that knowing this structure would be the biological equivalent to deciphering the Rosetta stone: the code would tell how the brain worked.

Many hormones of the body are 'peptides', designated as such because they are formed by ribbons of amino-acid peptides. The twenty 'essential' amino-acids in our bodies come together like the letters of an alphabet to form different peptide 'words'. Some peptides are short, formed by only three amino-acids, and fairly easy to untangle and reform.

The team in Aberdeen was quick to give its new brain opiate a name, 'enkephalin', and to recognize that it was a short peptide. But it was surprisingly difficult to untangle the individual amino-acids from one another. They enlisted the help of Howard Morris at Imperial College in London who, in a short time, was able to tell them that 'enkephalin' was really a mixture of two peptides each with five amino-acids. One was called 'met-enkephalin' and the other 'leu-enkephalin' because of the methionine in one and the leucine in the other.

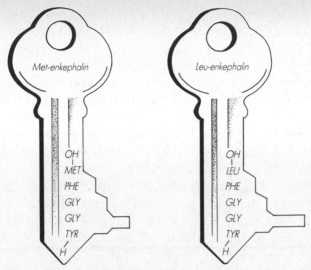

Fig. 11.3 Met-enkephaline and leu-enkephalin each contain five amino-acids

Other brain peptides had been discovered before. Indeed, two Nobel Prizes have been awarded for such discoveries, but in the earlier instances the brain peptides were directed from the brain to distant targets in the body. The significance of the discovery of the enkephalins rests in the realization that these brain hormones were destined for the brain; the presence of the opiate receptors within the brain made that a certainty.

Breaking this code established with certainty that the brain is a gland; the peptide sequence of enkephalin (see Fig. 11.3) verified that it was a 'peptide hormone' similar in every way to hormones that are formed by many glands in the body.

One of the best biochemists to study pituitary hormones was C. H. Li in San Francisco. From the pituitary he recovered 'prolactin' a hormone containing 199 amino-acids, and growth hormone, which contains 191 amino-acids. He found another peptide in the pituitary and called it 'lipotropin'. By 1965 the entire structure of lipotropin was discovered (see Fig. 11.4).

Lipotropin's structure was discovered a long time before anyone knew what it did, and the early notion that it regulated fat metabolism was quickly put away. By 1975 the sequence of lipotropin had been established in five different species. Always, its ninety-two peptides were arranged in much the same order.

None of those who had worked on the structure of lipotropin, a pituitary hormone, had connected it to enkephalin, the new brain hormone. But in 1975, at a conference in London, Derek Smythe

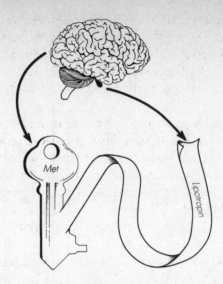

Fig. 11.4 Unravelling the structure of lipotropin made it clear that the brain and the pituitary were producing the same hormone

gave a seminar about lipotropin and showed slides of its amino-acid sequence. Embedded in the lipotropin sequence was the sequence of met-enkephalin.

This was evidence that the brain was making not only its own peptide hormones, but also hormones identical to those made by other glands. The questions that flowed after met-enkephalin, a brain hormone, was found in the pituitary gland are too numerous to recount. But most scientists correctly sensed that if the brain contained one pituitary hormone, it probably contained others. The brain was a gland, and the understanding of it would come by studying hormones, not electricity.

One of the first things scientists did was take a closer look at lipotropin. They discovered that a portion of this molecule, beta-endorphin, 'endorphin' for short, was an opiate quite similar to enkephalin. Even though it was bigger and found in different regions of the brain, endorphin was clearly a pituitary hormone with opiate-like qualities; it, too, would make the vas deferens contract.

In 1978 it was ascertained that lipotropin, a very big hormone, was only a fragment of an even larger molecule. In most laboratories, this giant is referred to by its weight alone; since it weighs 31,000 Daltons, it is called simply '31-K'.

This hormone, 31-K, is referred to as a 'pro-hormone', a large hormone that is made by the body and then cut into smaller parts.

No one understands why the body produces big molecules that must be broken down into smaller fragments before they can be useful, but pro-hormones are the rule, rather than the exception, in endocrinology. On the long ribbon of 31-K are several other hormones, each with a very distinct and different function (see Fig. 11.5).

Pro-hormones function much like the large Sunday edition of the *New York Times*: the printer finds it easiest to ship out all the sections together knowing that the readers will decide what they want. The fans will devour the sports pages, the bankers will read about finances, and the flat-hunters will pour through the tiny-print of the real estate ads. The body, in sending its endocrine signals from point to point, has employed this same communications strategy.

Soon after the discovery of 31-K, biochemists found another monstrously large peptide pro-hormone, this time in the adrenal gland in the abdomen, and called it '50-K'. Within its necklace-like arrangement of amino-acids was an even greater surprise – the repeating sequence of enkephalin, the 'brain' hormone that had begun the endocrine studies of the brain (see Fig. 11.6).

Knowing that both enkephalin and endorphin were opiate-like hormones, scientists looked more closely at the opiate receptor that had started the activity. They found several different kinds of opiate receptors but each, in a general way, was like a door with two key-holes, one arranged to be unlocked by endorphin and the other by enkephalin. The knowledge that one of the unlocking keys was stored in greatest quantity as 31-K in the pituitary gland and the other was stored in greatest quantity as 50-K in the adrenal gland was baffling: although the brain controls the release of both hormones, the tight capillaries in the brain limit the passage of these hormones into the brain.

In the cross-communication between opiate-smart endocrinologists and the electrically smart brain scientists, the mysteries of the gate-control theory of pain were discussed. As that phenomenon was taken into the endocrine laboratories, the fact that the brain was a gland, and that behaviour was modulated by hormones, became indisputable.

The endocrine explanation for the gate-control theory came from the employment of a procedure that is used virtually every day by drug companies searching for new and less-addicting pain-killers. It is called the 'tail-flick test'.

For this test, rats are housed in special cages that are not long enough for their tails, which protrude from the rear of the cage. A heating lamp is applied over the tail, which begins to 'flick' if the heat is uncomfortable. The temperature can be regulated precisely, and the tails are not burned in any way. Once in this device, rats are given drugs of different kinds to see if pain is perceived differently. Opium, for instance, would allow the rat to tolerate higher temperatures before the tail twitched. Any new synthetic drug can be tested in this way without risks to humans.

In 1969 the tail-flick test was employed to search for the location of the 'gates' within the brain. Stimulating electrodes were placed in various spots in the brains of rats housed in tail-flick cages. A spot was discovered in the middle of the brain that slammed gates closed. When this spot was stimulated, rats could feel no pain at all.

In 1976 Huda Akil, then in California, elected to repeat these remarkable experiments in animals that had been given naloxone, the opiate-receptor blocker. With naloxone on board, mid-brain stimulation had no effect; the rats felt every bit of pain. The pain relief that came from mid-brain stimulation did not come from electrically closed 'dry' gates alone. Since the benefit of the electric current had been blocked by naloxone, some opiate-like

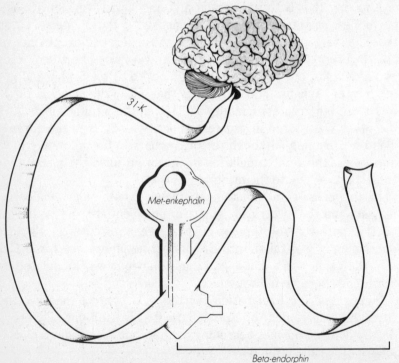

Fig. 11.5 31-K is a large pituitary molecule – a 'prohormone' – which contains the amino-acid sequences of many smaller hormones

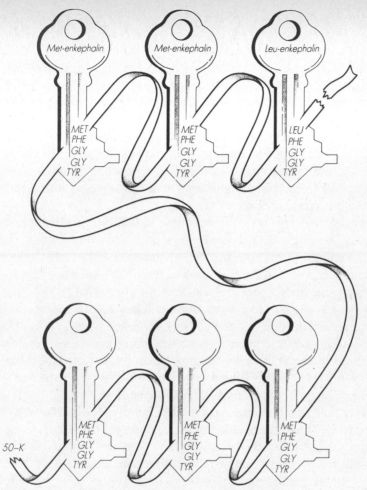

Fig. 11.6 50-K contains the repeating sequence of both met-enkephalin and leu-enkephalin and illustrates that opiate-like hormones are produced in the adrenal gland

hormone must have been released by the electrical stimulation. It was the hormone, not the electric current, that stopped the pain. Most likely, the opium released by mid-brain stimulation was coming from the brain itself.

This was a crucial bridging experiment that brought brain scientists away from the 'dry' electrical path of Galvani back to the 'wet' molecular path of Claude Bernard.

Only months later, this was verified in humans who were being treated with mid-brain stimulation for their pain: when stimulated, endorphin could be found in their spinal fluid, and the analgesic effects of their stimulation could be blocked by naloxone given before the stimulation.

Out of these serial experiments came two conclusions: opium is a hormone, and the brain is a gland that can make this hormone. The body also provides the brain with pain-killing drugs when the need arises; opiate-like hormones have been found in the gut, the pancreas, the gonads and white cells.

Enkephalin was the first brain hormone that was discovered in the brain's own pharmacy: endorphin was the second. Now, ten years later, scientists have found at least forty-five different brain hormones. There may be many more, but the principles seen in the opiate-like hormones are the same for every other hormone: they are released from one cell and trigger a response by interacting with a specific receptor on another cell.

Knowing that the opiate hormones, indeed all hormones, are scattered throughout the brain and body gives scientists the opportunity to 'intercept' the coded messages that are flowing between the two. Usually they look in the blood, knowing that the brain and the body speak to one another through that pipeline. Scientists know that the conversation will begin with the 'release' of a hormone from one cell and will be completed when another cell containing a receptor 'hears' the coded hormonal message. Like any conversation, it is easier to know the cells that are 'speaking', for they will release their messages. The cells that are 'listening' – receiving the codes – are more difficult to study.

The brain-to-body conversations that involve 31-K as the coded message are best understood. From these interceptions it has been established that the brain triggers the release of 31-K from the pituitary by first releasing two other hormones, vasopressin and 'corticotropin releasing factor' – for obvious reasons called 'CRF'. (These are the 'juices' that Hinsey postulated must flow from the brain to the pituitary.) When pituitary cells that produce 31-K 'hear' the coded message from the brain, they in turn release 31-K into the bloodstream.

Scientists know that pituitary cells will listen to a 'solo' by the brain (either juice alone – vasopressin or CRF – will release 31-K), but the cells respond much better if two substances (both juices: vasopressin and CRF) are sent to the pituitary at once. This phenomenon suggests that the brain does not sing 'solos' to the body, but 'harmonies'. Brain/body relationships might depend upon a chorus of individual hormones – perhaps fifty, perhaps five hundred – which are released together to sing hormonal harmonies to the body.

If the brain is communicating with the body in this manner, the decoding of a single 'solo' note will not be very helpful. Thus while more and more evidence supports the notion that hormones are the stuff of thought, it seems less likely that individual hormones control individual aspects of brain function. Combinations of hormones come together to do the brain's bidding.

It was assumed by Hinsey, Wislocki, du Vigneaud, and Harris, indeed by all neuroendocrinologists, that the hypothalamus converts the electrical signals of the brain into endocrine messages that can be carried to the body. The 31-K system shows this well: the greatest storehouse of it is in the pituitary; the greatest concentration of 31-K regulating hormones, vasopressin and CRF, is in the adjacent brain.

As anatomists have begun to look for the sites of production of 31-K, they have also looked for the presence of other brain hormones. To their surprise, they found vasopressin and CRF, which they had considered to be brain hormones, in many different glands of the body. This is perhaps best illustrated in the ovary and the gut: both vasopressin and CRF are found there. What is more surprising, cells that produce 31-K are also found in the ovary and the gut. Thus the entire combination of hormones of the 31-K system discovered in the brain is found in the abdomen – in the ovary and the gut. These organs manufacture not only their own 31-K but also the brain hormones that are responsible for its release (see Fig. 11.7).

Both vasopressin and 31-K fragments – 'ACTH' and 'MSH' – have been linked to memory. Researchers in Holland have shown this with such certainty in animals that synthetic preparations of these molecules are now being used to treat patients with loss of memory.

If memory springs from these hormones, does the ovary have memory? Can thinking go on outside the brain?

Before you dismiss this as madness, remember the disturbing conclusion that Karl Lashley (1890–1958) reached after looking for the 'site of memory' in the brain. For twenty years he had searched for the place in the brain where learning is stored by training rats to perform in a maze and then removing selective parts of the brain. Even though the brain operations produced all kinds of deficits of movement, the animals did not forget what they had learned; they could still find their way through the maze. He concluded: 'I sometimes feel in reviewing the evidence on localization of the memory trace that the necessary conclusion is that learning is not possible.'

Many psychologists since have speculated that memory must be stored in the body as photographic information is stored in a holo-

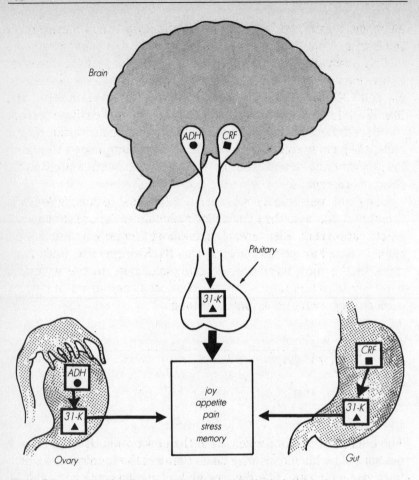

Fig. 11.7 The release of 31-K from the pituitary is controlled by the brain

gram. They contend that there is no single site in the brain for the 'piano lessons' and another site for the 'French lessons'. They say that memory is diffused everywhere and focused nowhere.

If memory is dependent upon hormones and if memory is holographic, finding the hormones of memory in many sites outside the brain moves the 'engram for memory' that Lashley was searching for outside the brain.

Many glandular organs, however, can produce an electrical signal that is carried from one cell to the next. Finding electricity in the endocrine system unites the brain and the endocrine system in the reverse direction. As certainly as hormones have found their way into the brain, electricity has found its way into the endocrine system. If electricity, produced by combinations of hormones in the brain, can carry messages from the brain to the body, cannot electricity, produced by hormones in the body, carry messages to the brain?

The ovary and the gut have all the machinery for a 'private' endocrine conversation; they produce the same juices – vasopressin and CRF – that the brain produces, and they make 31-K just like the pituitary. Although scientists might not easily intercept the coded messages that flow between individual ovarian or gut cells, they know that the machines of the mind, indeed the same brain hormones, are present in the ovary, the gut and predictably many more organs.

The giant molecule 31-K is specifically linked to specific kinds of 'thoughts', more so than any other molecule and more so than any electrical current. Pleasure, pain, memory, appetite and stress are each modified in specific ways by tiny 31-K fragments. Each fragment of the molecule becomes one 'solo' note in the hormonal harmony of thought, but if these solo notes come from the ovary, does not the ovary contribute to thought?

Shoreline of Wonder

The philosophical consequences of the new notion that the mind is modulated by hormones may be as great as the medical and scientific consequences. The double-think of modern science – 'Molecules shape the body, but electricity shapes the mind' – ends abruptly with the realization that regulatory hormones control both brain and body functions.

Since Plato's description of the shadows on a cave, philosophers have held that something outside the body shapes thoughts. Descartes's dualism is the best example of this; his world was cut horizontally in half. Above his dividing plane, events were ruled by spiritual laws. Below that plane, events were governed by physical laws. In Descartes's scheme, the pineal gland protruded up into the spiritual world like a lightning rod that carried the soul into the body. Although modern intellectuals do not share his view of the pineal, his dualism lingers in the corners of many minds.

The belief that the brain was driven by electricity has been an important factor in the longevity of Descartes's dualism. Electricity obviously came from above – Franklin's kite experiments proved that. Moreover, it had the invisible, mystical qualities of a spirit. But to understand the importance of brain electricity to modern Western thought, consider again the right/left split of human brain functions.

The left brain thinks serially; it considers one thing at a time – a letter, word or number. Ideas must be reduced to letters and words, and quantities must be reduced to numbers. Reduction is the very essence of left-brain thought processing; to enter the left brain's thinking machinery, a thing must be reduced to something smaller than itself. These reductions must be kept separate and at a given instant, in reading, writing, listening, or speaking, the left brain must focus on one reduction.

By contrast, the right brain is committed to patterns. All that it does involves wholeness. The right brain always considers the whole of something and, at any given moment, the right brain must focus on many interrelated things.

The very nature of electricity dovetails with left-brain function: electrical currents do flow serially. Electrical sparks, or smaller electrons, must remain isolated one from another as thoughts are isolated in the left brain; the electrical signals that are employed in communications devices such as radios, telephones, televisions, and computers must be dealt with one at a time very much like the left brain focuses on one reduction at a time.

At the time that Descartes's notion that the pineal was the seat of the soul was held to be absurd, another kind of spirit, one formed from electricity and measurable on the surface of the brain and individual nerves, was enthroned in the brain. The essence of human life, the conscious 'me', was assigned an electrical quality and placed in the part of the brain that communicates serially: the left brain. An Aristotlean hierarchy of organs was allowed, which assigned the left brain the highest place, gave electricity the highest function and gave reductionistic thoughts the highest priority.

With all of this, the right brain was thought of as sub-human; those mystics, often from the East, who espoused non-verbal, holistic, mystical thoughts were regarded as lesser intellectuals.

The new hormone-based paradigm for the mind acknowledges that electricity does flow from nerve to nerve and can be measured on the surface of the brain or on the membranes of individual nerves. But these superficial signals are little more than dry echoes of deeper molecular events going on within the cell.

Scientists now believe that the mind will be best comprehended by focusing on intracellular molecular events, rather than on superficial electrical signals. Although this is a new paradigm, nearly all of the early experiments demonstrate that regulatory hormones join in holistic patterns that may be understood by organs other than the brain. The mechanisms of the mind are thus released from the conceptual confines of the reductionistic left brain. The mechanisms that drive thought are found all over the body and, wherever they live, they function at their highest level by recognizing the molecular patterns of the combination of hormones that modulate thought.

As scientists accept this new paradigm, the primary mechanisms of intelligent thought must be viewed differently. The mind is made pattern dependent and comes to share in the ubiquitous secret of evolutionary survival: pattern recognition.

Pattern recognition is the *sine qua non* of the genetic code, of the DNA/RNA interactions, which provide the blueprints for life; pattern recognition underlies all immunology – the antigen-antibody reactions that recognize and defend 'self'; pattern recognition is basic to all the hormone/hormone receptor interactions of cell regulation; and pattern recognition is the highest form of thought. It is the synchrony, the synergism and the spatial juxtaposition of whirling hormonal forces that give life to the human soul.

Is this molecular maelstrom divine? I think so: it creates life, it is ubiquitous, it cannot be broken apart, it cannot be contained, it cannot be copied, it is eternal.

Arthur Koestler observed that scientific reductions have led to a divorce of reason and faith. The ultimate reduction is a bleak and faithless formula, $E=MC^2$; it has placed mankind on the brink of global self-destruction and created a spiritual ice age. The new view of the mind may lead to the rapprochement between faith and reason, for it seems certain that an unknowable 'force' gives life to the molecules of the mind.

Other formulae, espousing harmonious, symmetrical, beautiful, creative and joyful patterns, may lead mankind away from the threat of nuclear war, but it seems certain that these patterns will only be comprehended by minds which understand that holistic thought is the human brain's highest evolutionary accomplishment and, without doubt, the best guide to evolutionary survival.

12

*I*n 1797, forty years before the cell theory, Xavier Bichat (1771–1802) proposed that the work of the body was systematically divided: the bones came together to form the skeletal system, the esophagus, stomach and bowels came together to form the digestive system, the trachea and lungs formed the respiratory system, and so on. Bichat divided the body into twenty-one such systems, but modern biologists acknowledge only the nervous, skeletal, cardio-vascular, digestive, respiratory, muscular, immune, lymphatic, reproductive, genito-urinary, blood, skin and endocrine systems. In this decade a new system, the paracrine system, was discovered.

The nervous system was recognized long ago, but the endocrine system is very recent. Both the nervous system and the endocrine system are regulatory systems, and the work that they do might be equated to office work. These are the white-collar systems of the body. Historians describing the discovery of the paracrine system might equate it to an industry-like 'takeover'. The paracrine system centralizes the two management teams, the old nervous system and the new endocrine system. In this merger we see a new and different kind of management style that directs the management teams out of their offices into the factory-sites of the body. The paracrine management philosophy assigns regulatory hormones to the site of work: gut managers reside in the gut, kidney managers live in the kidney, and blood vessel managers are stationed in blood vessels, and so on.

It was the recent development of hormone-specific stains that allowed scientists to see the hormone-laden regulatory cells that are scattered about the body. Many scientists feel that the paracrine system, or its equivalent, is the oldest in biology, pointing to the presence of regulating hormones even in the earliest of single-cell evolutionary animals to prove their point.

Most people are not aware of the paracrine system, yet the term is about forty-five years old. It was introduced in 1938 by Friedrich Feytrer (1895–1973), a pathologist in Danzig, to describe his observation that some hormones are carried from one cell directly to a neighbouring cell, the 'parallel cell', hence the name 'paracrine system'. In 1966, a British biologist, A.G.E. Pearse, called attention again to endocrine cells that were scattered about in surprising places. But not until hormones were found in the brain was the significance of paracrine management understood. With Roger Guillemin's Nobel acceptance speech in 1978, paracrinology entered the everyday vocabulary of scientists. The term is a biological portmanteau that describes a host of biological events involving both the nervous system and the endocrine system. In one surprising link, the brain to the testicles, many of the principles of paracrinology become evident.

Many centuries before people were performing surgery on humans, they were operating on animals. Crude operations were performed with the intent of modifying behaviour. Testicles, for example, have been removed from horny, rapacious males to tame them for at least 5,000 years.

In 1771 Hunter elected to do the reverse and add the male testicle to a female animal. In this simple experiment Hunter confirmed that the brain behaved like a gland. Hunter's observation is what paracrinology is all about: regulating hormones modulate or control the function of an organ. Although Hunter first saw it in the brain, it is the rule for every organ.

In the early part of the last century, a curious link between the brain and the testicles was again described. Two French phrenologists described shrinkage of the left cerebellum if the right testicle was removed, or vice versa – right cerebellum and left testicle. What was just as remarkable, if the left cerebellum was damaged, the right testicle became smaller.

In 1959 a Hungarian anatomist, Janos Szentagothai, described similar structural changes in brain cells after removing endocrine glands – the ovary, testicle, or adrenal – and presented convincing evidence that there was a two-way street between one side of the brain and glands on the other side of the body. Szentagothai's laboratory has been working on these relationships steadily since that time, and his team has confirmed that lesions in tiny areas of the left brain will limit growth of glands on the right, and vice versa. Scientists working with Szentagothai have also found shrunken brain cells in the same area of the left brain if the right glands are removed (see Fig. 12.1). These changes are not the result of the

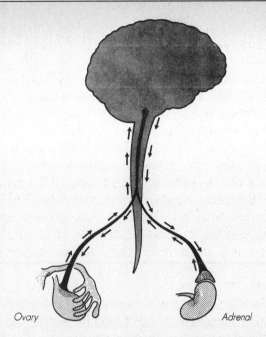

Fig. 12.1 Direct connections exist between the glands of the body and the brain

hormonal messages that are carried by the bloodstream because they have been noted in animals that do not have a pituitary.

Few brain scientists paid much attention to these brain-to-testicle links; they did not fit with the paradigm that the brain is electrically driven. Nor did they dovetail with Wislocki's view of the neuroendocrine system, which regarded the pituitary as a necessary link between the brain and the endocrine system.

The team in Hungary stuck to its belief and now scientists are forced to concede that the observations are fundamentally correct. Sophisticated endocrine tests of the brain demonstrate that the brain is changed, it 'thinks' differently, if the gonads are removed.

The significance of this link is immense; it demonstrates that messages are carried from the brain to the endocrine system and from the endocrine system to the brain within nerves. These messages are not electrical but molecular. The coded signals move down nerves from the brain to the glands to nourish hormone-producing cells, and molecules move up nerves from the glands to the brain to nourish thought-producing cells.

Regulatory messages or hormones flow from specific regions of the brain to specific glands within 'hollow' nerve fibres exactly as Erasistratus, Galen and Descartes had taught.

The science of neuroendocrinology – the brain-to-pituitary link that was discerned by Hinsey, Wislocki, du Vigneaud, and Harris – is dependent upon hormones flowing within nerve axons. This phenomenon, axonal flow, was first noted by Ernst and Barta Scharrer, who suggested that hormone 'managers' were being sent by the brain to peripheral organs through nerve fibres. For many decades it was assumed that axonal flow was always 'down', that is, it moved away from the brain.

In the past decade it has become clear that hormones also move 'up' nerve fibres from the body to the brain. This was noted using many different experimental techniques: hormones injected into the eye are carried back to the brain, tracers injected into the tongue are carried back to the brainstem and, most remarkably, substances injected into the thigh muscle may be carried into the spinal cord. The best-studied such molecule is 'nerve growth factor'.

Nerve growth factor was discovered about twenty years ago: it is made in many places but chiefly in the salivary glands. It is carried as a hormone in the bloodstream to the endings of nerves and sucked up into the nerve in the way that an elephant trunk sucks up water. Once in the nerve, it is carried on special intracellular barges several feet back towards the nervous system, where it nourishes special kinds of nerves. If the trunk-like nerve is pinched in any way, the central nerve cell will die. Moreover, if antibodies are injected into the bloodstream, the circulating nerve growth factor is destroyed and, as a result, the central cells that depend upon nerve growth factor will die of starvation (see Fig. 12.2).

Molecules that have no biological function but can be traced wherever they travel are called 'tracers'. One of the best tracers is an extract of horseradish that can be injected into living cells without ill effects. Injection of this material, horseradish peroxidase, into different glands has demonstrated 'retrograde transport pathways' very similar to those suggested by Szentagothai's experiments. Similar pathways have also been found from organs that are not thought of as glands. If this tracer is injected into the stomach, for example, it can be recovered in very specific regions of the brain. If it is injected into a leg muscle, it appears in the spinal cord. If it is sprayed into the nose, it appears in the brain's olfactory tract (see Fig. 12.3).

Molecules move not only from the brain to the endocrine system but also from the endocrine system, indeed, from all parts of the body to the brain.

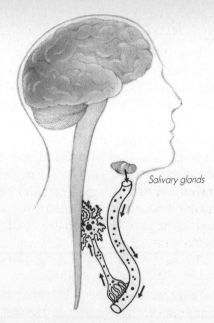

Fig. 12.2 Nerve growth factor is made in the salivary glands and makes its way into the bloodstream, where it is carried backwards up the nerve as food for nerves near the spinal cord

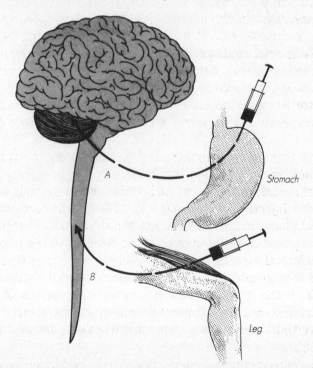

Fig. 12.3 Horseradish peroxidase is a powerful 'tracer': injected into a leg muscle, it is carried backwards into the spinal cord; injected into the stomach, it is carried into the brain

Scientists can take the nucleus out of a single cell from the inner cheek of a green frog and transplant it into the egg of a brown frog. In a few days the identical twin of the green frog pops out of the brown frog's egg. If scientists took out a thousand-cell nucleii from one green frog and transplanted it in this way, they could produce a thousand identical green twins. This is called 'cloning'. In every cell in your body is the genetic code for your entire body. By transplanting the cell nucleus into an egg, you could replicate yourself, billions of times, if you wished, and every one of your cloned children would be your identical twin.

Cloning emphasizes that each cell in the body contains enough information to produce an entire brain and endocrine system. Knowing this, the production of regulating hormones by paracrine cells becomes more credible.

Every organ is a hormone-producing gland. Jesse Roth, an American endocrinologist, believes that every regulatory peptide can be made everywhere. Although 'glands' produce the greatest quantities of regulatory hormones and store them for sudden release, paracrine hormones are found virtually everywhere in the body.

A single cell may be commissioned by the larger society of cells – the society first described by Virchow – to produce a single molecule. Such a cell will first switch on the genes in its nucleus that carry the instructions for such production.

If a gene in the cell nucleus is switched on, its DNA ribbons will split apart and allow a xerox-like copy of its code to be made. The copy is formed from RNA. Like a precious manuscript that is not allowed to leave a library, DNA molecules are not allowed to leave the confines of the cell's nucleus; only RNA molecules – the xerox copies – can do that.

During most of the past thirty years, the period of the revolution in molecular biology, it was assumed that the brain could control the release of substances from the surface of the cell. But in the past few years scientists have come to believe that the switching-on of genes may also be controlled by the brain.

This may be best explained by looking closely at muscle or, more specifically, at the 'dark' and 'white' meat of a turkey. White muscle is involved in quick activities such as wing movement. Dark muscle is involved in slow movement such as walking and standing. If the nerves that go to fast and slow muscles are switched – the nerves destined to control the wings switched with those destined to control the legs – the muscles that move the wings become slow and those that move the legs become fast. Although scientists have not yet determined what it is that switches on the genes that produce slow muscle instead of fast muscle, most of the evidence suggests that this message, which comes from the brain, is hormonal not electrical. These brain hormones may move into the very centre of the cell, the nucleus, and modify the genes that control it.

Only in the past year have scientists been able to see a switched-on gene; the method, devised by John Coghlan in Melbourne, is called 'hybridization histochemistry'. This technique allows you to look at the coded RNA that the cell has sent into the cytoplasm, that is, at the xerox copies of the genes. Such RNA will only be in the cytoplasm if the gene has been switched on. Hybridization histochemistry will allow scientists to untangle the puzzle of the 'dark' and 'white' meat, and many similar puzzles, and thereby understand the role that the brain plays in genetic regulation.

Central to the paradigm that the mind is modulated by hormones is the recognition that the stuff of thought is not caged in the brain but is scattered all over the body; regulatory hormones are ubiquitous. Gone are the days when scientists believed one hormone was made by one gland. Insulin, for example, may be made in greatest quantity in the pancreas, but it is made in other surprising places, like the brain, and even by tiny one-cell organisms without a pancreas. The parameceum, for example, makes insulin as do many other small animals that do not have a pancreas.

Roth has proposed that every regulating hormone can be produced everywhere in the body, and the cloning experiments of genetic engineers underscore the feasibility of this. The new science of paracrinology extends Roth's observation by noting that these regulating hormones are not static; they move from cell to cell, indeed, from organ to organ. Moreover, their movement lacks a predetermined direction; to-and-fro movement is the rule not the exception.

Untangling these relationships will be much more difficult than untangling the electrical circuits of the brain. There are more places to look, more things to look for and more directions that signals might take. Looking for a tiny circuit in the brain or looking for a single opiate-like hormone in the brain both involved needle-in-the-haystack kinds of searches, but nearly every paracrine relationship that warrants untangling involves currents of hormones that flow between cells, in the bloodstream and nerve fibres. At every level the movement of the regulating hormones is bidirectional, compounding the difficulty of the untangling effort.

The magnitude of the puzzle is increased further by the realization that regulatory peptides may do different things for different organs, even in the same species. The hormone insulin, for example, performs sugar management for the body but does quite another thing in the brain: injected into the brain of baboons it modifies their behaviour. At the moment it appears to be the best 'slimming' hormone that exists, but for that function to be realized it must be fed to the brain, not the body.

To compound things, many hormone-controlled activities depend upon pulsatile secretion. The best example of this is the control of egg release from the ovary: neither a single injection nor a continuous infusion of the responsible brain hormones works well. Six or eight injections, interspersed at regular intervals over several hours, are necessary for 'controlled' ovulation. Scientists predict that many brain-controlled body functions depend upon similar well-timed, pulsatile bursts of hormonal harmonies from the brain.

Now paracrinology's biggest surprise: glandular cells 'turn over', that is, when a hormone-producing cell dies, a new cell will appear in its place. But for more than a century it has been assumed that brain cells – neurones – do not turn over. Scientists claimed that nature planted billions of neurones in the brain at birth, but as the years passed the number of these cells diminished. Some experts said that many million neurones died each day, never to be replaced. But in 1984 came the solid experimental evidence that brain cells, like gland cells, turn over; new neurones are being produced in the brain all the time.

Learning about neuronal turnover is a scientific activity that has just begun, but even at the beginning one sees that the fabric of the mind has been given new mystery. How does a dying neurone pass its information to its replacement? Is there some ten command-ment-like tablet, chiselled into the genetic code, which is swal-lowed by the new cell and then replicated like a gene? Does that cell, on its death, pass the same information in the same way? If a new brain cell can swallow such a tablet produced by a dying brain cell, can it swallow other tablets produced by other cells? Can the brain, like a muscle that is exercised, grow new cells that will make it stronger; or conversely, does the unexcercised brain atrophy much as a muscle withers away if it is unused?

It is unlikely that scientists will untangle paracrinology's Gordian knot tomorrow or even in this century. Few biological processes are as complex as those in paracrinology, yet no other aspect of biology could bring an equivalent good to humankind.

Since the time of Aristotle brain scientists have been trying to label the stuff of thought; first it was quintessence, then a humour, then animal spirit, then electricity and, most recently, hormones.

As brain hormones are placed at the top of the hierarchy of mind-stuff, what will be the new driving force?

It is too early to tell. Both laboratory workers and clinicians, especially psychiatrists and psychologists, are silent on the issue. Both groups are sophisticated historians who note that the religious, philosophical and social consequences of the driving force may be of greater importance than the stuff of thought. They are appropriately cautious.

The wisest brain scientists seem to be watching the physicists who know most about the elementary particles in atoms. As they listen to physicists describe electrons, neutrons and protons as 'forces', not 'matter', they wonder if brain hormones may also be a force rather than a substance.

Brain scientists hear physicists say that a single electron, spinning about a central atomic nucleus, may change orbits by a mechanism that knows no time and space. These events compel physicists to believe that 'forces', not matter, are the fundamental building blocks of nature. They claim that the parts of the atom that artists draw as concrete orbiting balls are not substantial things at all, but forces; physicists say you are totally composed of these atomic forces and have no real substance.

What do physicists believe is the stuff of matter? In two words: interdependent forces. One physicist, Ervin Schrodinger, wrote a now-famous essay to demonstrate to brain scientists that these forces are of fundamental importance to brain function and provide the stuff of thought a mysterious link to the stuff of matter. To prove his point, he described a theoretical experiment in which a cat was placed in a box with a force detector that would trigger a device to kill the cat. If the cat were left alone it would live, but Schrodinger demonstrated that the mere contemplation of the experiment by an outside viewer would drain some 'force' from the box. If the force detector were fine-tuned to measure this loss, then trigger the death device, the cat would die. This now legendary experiment demonstrates that the stuff of matter and the stuff of thought are both interdependent forces.

Although Schrodinger's experiment suggests that physicists understand how all of the physical forces of the world are intertwined, nothing could be further from the truth. Three of the four primary forces – strong interactions, weak interactions, and electromagnetism – have well-documented interrelationships; the fourth force, gravity, is not at all understood and cannot be related to the other forces. Scientists believe that the discovery of a fifth force, the unifying force, will explain gravity and show that all the physical forces are related by ubiquitous, fundamental principles.

As gravity is the great unknown of physics, memory is the great enigma of brain science.

To those brain scientists committed to the paradigm of an electrically driven brain, memory is often described by using computer-like terms such as 'reverberating circuits' or 'cybernetics'. To the new breed of scientist committed to the paradigm of a hormonally driven brain, memory has a pattern-dependent molecular structure. The first paradigm is based on the physical principles of the electromagnetic force. The second paradigm, depending upon molecular interactions, invokes that force but also the forces of strong interactions and weak interactions, which hold molecules together. Neither of these competing paradigms invokes the fourth force, gravity. Memory may be like gravity. And its understanding may not come until the fifth, unifying force, is comprehended.

Consider an experiment performed by Hunter more than 200 years ago. Stag antlers, Hunter knew, grow more rapidly than any other biological tissue and always at the same time of the year. It is the rapid elongation of the antlers while in 'velvet' that has led to the centuries-old view that wafer-thin slices of velvet serve as an effective male aphrodiasiac; to this day the sale of these wafers is a multi-million dollar business in the Orient.

Hunter elected to divide the blood supply to one half of the stag's skull just at the time that the antlers were scheduled to begin their rapid growth. Only the antler with its blood supply intact grew, proving that blood supply was important to growth. But within a fortnight, after a new blood supply had grown into the skull, the stunted antler began to grow. Hunter was then able to watch a minor miracle: the growth pattern of the new antler was the absolute mirror-image of the previously formed antler – it had the same length and the same number of tines, but was a perfect reversal.

Hunter was clever enough to ask, 'What force guides this growth?' In all other body systems 'tropisms' are expected. A developing nerve, for example, is drawn towards an already-

developed muscle. But in the case of the antler, the perfectly symmetrical growth is without any 'tropic' influence. The molecules
forming the bone have a life of their own and somehow, as they
reach towards the sky, carry within them a pattern for antler
formation, not an identical pattern but a mirror-image. How could
the molecules possibly know they were on the right side of the head
and not the left? Hunter only posed the question. It is a question
that cannot be answered by any of today's biologists or physicists,
and it neatly underscores the ignorance of us all.

The miracle of the antler, like the miracle of gravity and
memory, demands a new 'force' of some kind – a unifying force. It
is not explained by any of the four forces that the physicists talk
about; neither brain hormones nor brain electricity can move
cleverly into 'nothingness'.

Wise men from India predicted that mystical forces regulated
the activities of the brain and the body. Inherent in much of what
they taught was the notion that the body can be taught to 'think'.
Paracrinology verifies their view: the chemical machinery that
produces rational thought rests within the body and outside the
brain. It is this view of the stuff of thought that provides those in
the East a respect for karma – the mysterious life-giving force that
flows from life to life. Their view of karma is in every way like the
modern physicists view of electrons. They say it is not 'matter' but
a 'force'. The Hindu commitment to reincarnation is a wager that
karma moves from one moving life to another moving life by the
same 'magic' that moves atomic electrons between orbits.

With the discovery of the non-substantial nature of atomic particles and the prediction of a unifying force, Western science has
validated much of the ancient, holistic wisdom written 5,000 years
ago in vedic scriptures. The karma of the Eastern mind is so similar
to the interdependent forces that scientists such as Schrodinger
claim are both the stuff of matter and the stuff of thought that yogis
might rightly claim that karma does exist because Western science
has proved it.

The reductionists in the West, however, cannot accept the holistic wisdom of Eastern mysticism even though, at the most fundamental level, their own tools have verified it, and their best physicists are committed to the conceptual need for a unifying force that
defies reduction.

13

Why is the Brain Hollow?

Fig. 13.1 shows an X-ray of the 'ventricles', formed by injecting a dye into the hollow, fluid-filled centre of a brain. All
animals have an inner fluid-filled space. But why?

Most teachers would say something like this. The brain is so soft
that it must float. If it were not floating in water, you couldn't turn
somersaults or play rough-and-tumble football without damaging
your jelly-like brain. The brain keeps a cushion of water inside
itself and another cushion of water outside itself so that it is doubly
protected from forceful injuries.

Most scientists believe that water enters the ventricles – the
fluid-filled centre – through the 'choroid plexus', a structure that
resembles a bunch of grapes and waves in the waters of the ventricle. They also believe this water flows out of the ventricles into
the 'sub-arachnoid space'. They would tell you that water then
flows around the brain and returns into the venous circulation
through other grape-like structures, the 'Paccionian granulations',
which hang into large veins at the top of the head.

The neatly integrated paradigm for brain water shown in
Fig. 13.2 was derived from experiments done by Walter Dandy in
Baltimore in 1911. It is one of the most frequently produced
diagrams in science and medicine and has been reproduced in the
best textbooks of neuroanatomy, neurophysiology, psychiatry,
neurology and neurosurgery. As these complex water-flow pathways are not easily described, I will refer to them as the 'Dandy
paradigm'.

Most brain scientists and brain physicians honour the Dandy
paradigm as a navigator honours the North Star. The arrows he
drew for water-flow have guided many different kinds of thoughts
about the brain since the day he drew them, yet new scientific
evidence makes it difficult, if not impossible, to accept these guid-

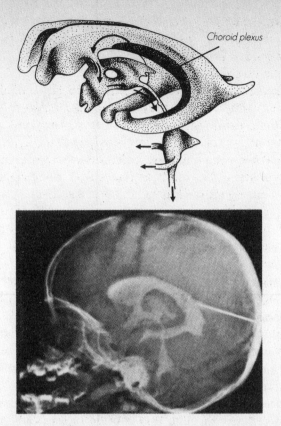

Choroid plexus

Fig. 13.1 Leonardo's cast of the ventricles formed by injecting white plastic into the sub-arachnoid space which surrounds the brain

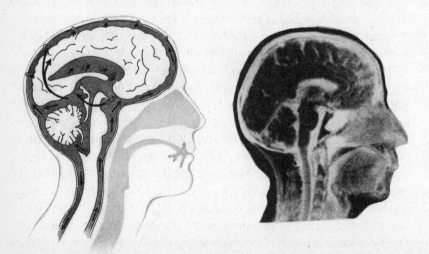

Fig. 13.2 *Left*: Once water escapes from the ventricles, it flows over the surface of the brain. *Right*: The scan shows the fluid-filled space around the brain

ing arrows any longer. It is a mismeme; the experimental facts no longer allow it to be 'true', and we need a paradigm switch.

To understand Dandy's mismeme and its passage into the heads of scientific teachers, let us go back to Galen.

In the second century Galen performed rather complicated brain surgery on living unanaesthetized animals that were strapped to boards. He describes the removal of different portions of the brain in animals with vivid detail and an accuracy that convinces me that he did what he says he did. He notes the changes in brain volume caused by respiration exactly as I have seen them countless times in humans during brain surgery. In his dissections Galen describes the right and left cerebral ventricles, the midline third ventricle and the aqueduct that connects the third to the fourth ventricle beneath the cerebellum.

Galen gave the different ventricles well-defined functions even though there was no reason at all to link them to function. He said that new ideas were generated in the right and left lateral ventricles and that they were stored as memories in the midline chamber of the third ventricle. What did the fourth ventricle do? It was the chamber of wisdom and judgement. This view was unquestioned for at least 1,500 years.

In AD 1500 Leonardo filled the ventricles of the brain with molten wax to form the first cast of the ventricle. From these he produced the first accurate drawings of it, but he did not question the universal belief that highest intellectual thoughts resided mysteriously in these spaces.

The elegant art work of Vesalius emphasized that the human brain was hollow. But this hollowness did not excite much interest because it was assumed that animal spirit in the brain was a liquid that needed storage somewhere before it was pushed out into the nerves. Descartes's drawings of the ventricles were crude and wrong, but he made the waterworks in these spaces dovetail with his anatomically linked philosophy. His clever placement of the seat of the soul in the pineal, just above and between the chamber of memory and the chamber of wisdom and judgement, attests again to the chicanery of his blend of mechanics and philosophy.

To Galen, Leonardo, Vesalius and Descartes, the ventricles were cavities that stored the animal spirit that moved muscles.

Dissections performed in 1768 in Hunter's laboratory found lymphatics, the tiny, gossamer-thin tubules that carry lymph back to the heart from most regions of the body. He and his brother William Hunter called the network the 'second circulation'. Before their dissections, it was believed that every organ in the body received an artery, a vein and a nerve. The discovery of the lymphatics by the Hunter brothers gave every organ a fourth kind of tubular linkage.

But Hunter was careful enough to note that the brain did not have its own lymphatics. Instead, it was filled with ventricular fluid. He postulated that the lymph of the brain was carried from it by the interconnected inner ventricles. Noting that the third ventricle was connected to the pituitary gland by a funnel, the 'infundibulum', he postulated that brain lymph was carried into the pituitary, which he assumed to be a lymph gland. Hunter made these deductions before microscopic studies of cells were possible and there was no reason to believe from observation that the pituitary gland was any different from lymph glands elsewhere.

For the entire nineteenth century the brain was considered to be a giant electrical network. The brain biologists of that period were content to accept Hunter's notion that brain water moved into the ventricles and then out of the brain by way of the pituitary. The paradigm kept the brain relatively 'dry', all the better for the electrical circuits of the brain.

Hunter's paradigm equating brain ventricular fluid to lymph was accepted until 1871. In that year, pituitary tumours were first found in human giants by Pierre Marie. He assumed that such tumours allowed an accumulation of lymph in the brain, and that brain lymph, in turn, caused gigantic growth. Not until the birth of endocrinology in 1902 did scientists question Hunter's notion that the ventricles and the pituitary together drained the brain of its lymph. By 1908 it became clear that the pituitary gland was the master gland of the body and secreted a substance, growth hormone, which caused animals to grow. Cushing suggested in that year that excessive secretion of growth hormone from the pituitary, not the accumulation of brain lymph within the ventricle, caused gigantism.

Since Cushing had given the pituitary another function totally unrelated to the lymphatic function assigned to it by Hunter, the ventricles were quite suddenly left with no known function. The question, 'Why is the brain hollow?', then was unquestionably not transparent; it had a significance equal to the question, 'Why is the heart hollow?', which had stimulated Harvey. Dandy, one year out of medical school, sought an answer.

Dandy had decided as a medical undergraduate that he wanted to be a brain surgeon. In those days, this meant that he would spend several years as a general surgeon with Dr Halsted and then extra time in neurosurgical training. When he did his experiments on the hollow brain, he had had no surgical training. He had not even begun his general surgical training, but he performed neuro-surgical procedures on animals that even by today's standards are very difficult technically.

Dandy's experiments were performed in dogs and were designed to learn more about the disease of 'hydrocephalus'; in those days, before antibiotics, meningitis was commonplace and those who survived were often left with 'water on the brain' or hydrocephalus. The understanding of hydrocephalus, he reasoned, would lead to an answer to the question, 'Why is the brain hollow?'

In Dr Halsted's general surgical practice, operations for obstructed stomachs and obstructed bladders were commonplace and, as a medical student, Dandy could not have escaped the lesson that 'outlet obstruction' caused ballooning of hollow organs.

Dandy quite naturally asked, 'Could outlet obstruction cause the ballooned-up ventricles of hydrocephalus?' and designed experi-ments to test that possibility. In dogs, he placed a 'cork' in the aqueduct that linked the third and fourth ventricles (see Fig. 13.3).

After this operation the ventricles were much larger, very simi-lar to those seen in hydrocephalus. To Dandy, this development meant that the ventricles had been blown up like a balloon as a consequence of outlet obstruction.

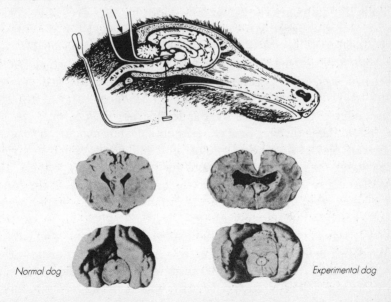

Normal dog   Experimental dog

Fig. 13.3 Dandy put a cork in the aqueduct behind the third ventricle in a dog's brain, noticed that the ventricles grew larger and concluded that hydrocephalus was a disease of 'outlet obstruction'

Dandy's next question, 'Where could the water come from?', also prompted a direct experimental approach. He opened one half of the brain, the left cerebrum, like a clam in order to remove the choroid plexus that lay in the floor of the ventricle. Then he inserted his 'cork' in the aqueduct as he had done before. Now he found that only the right ventricle became swollen, the one that still contained the choroid plexus.

Dandy concluded that the water in the ventricles that caused hydrocephalus came from the choroid plexus. It appeared to him that water was continually coming from the choroid plexus and needed to get out of the brain. If it could not pass through the outlets, the brain would swell like a balloon, in every way like the stomach and the bladder.

Dandy was assuming that the water in the brain was not important. His focus on intraventricular water was in keeping with the times: everyone assumed that the brain was driven by electricity. Physics, not chemistry, was important to the brain. In looking at the inside of the brain as a balloon, Dandy was able to eschew all chemical considerations and base his paradigm on physics and, in this instance, on the laws of fluid mechanics. His paradigm was based on the premise that the water in the ventricles had no chemical relationship to the electrically driven surrounding brain.

Next Dandy asked, 'Where does the water go once it leaves the brain?' To find out, he opened up both the right and left side of the skull, lifted up both the left and the right hemispheres of the brain and passed a gauze strip around the mid brain. He had hoped to demonstrate that this manoeuvre also caused hydrocephalus. But it didn't. After this procedure, the ventricles were normal in size. He repeated the experiment, but on this second occasion he soaked the gauze strips in tincture of iodine to induce a scar. After this procedure, the ventricles were indeed larger than before.

From these three sets of experiments, Dandy concluded that the choroid plexus was the source of ventricular water; that ventricular water passed out of the brain; and that once outside the brain, ventricular water flowed around the brain to the veins at the top of the skull where it re-entered the circulation. These experiments gave birth to the Dandy paradigm.

Very quickly Dandy gave his experiments clinical significance. He concluded that there were two kinds of hydrocephalus. One kind resulted from blockade of the aqueduct: fluid could not get out of the ventricle. For such patients he proposed a diverting operation that allowed the fluid produced in the choroid plexus to leak out of the brain through a new surgically constructed hole in the floor of the third ventricle. This operation became known as a 'third ventriculostomy' (see Fig. 13.4).

The second kind of hydrocephalus resulted from infectious post-meningitic scars around the surface of the brain. Fluid could get out of the brain, but it could not make its way to the veins at the top of the head. For such patients, Dandy proposed another kind of operation: removal of the choroid plexus, the source of the offending fluid (see Fig. 13.5).

Dandy did many of these operations on patients, and for two decades other surgeons all over the world followed in his footsteps. But a host of retrospective statistical analyses of these operations demonstrate that neither choroid plexectomy nor third ventriculostomy was an effective treatment for hydrocephalus.

With the development of malleable plastics in World War II, 'shunts' of many types were developed, and now hundreds of these operations are performed daily throughout the world to treat hydrocephalus. The upper tip of the shunt is typically placed in the ventricle, usually the right, and the distal end is placed in the

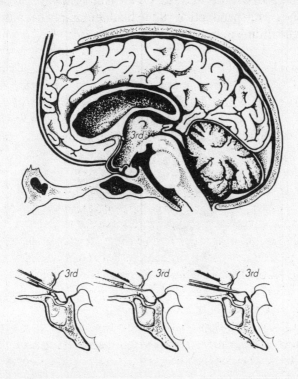

Fig. 13.4 Convinced that water entered the ventricle through the choroid plexus and moved through the ventricular system, Dandy deduced that diseases that blocked the aqueduct would cause hydrocephalus

abdomen; this allows fluid from the ventricle to drain into the abdomen (see Fig. 13.6).

There are many technical problems with shunts: children may outgrow them, the tubing may kink, break, twist, become plugged with debris or become infected. But the operation is one that is generally quite successful; it has made hydrocephalus a manageable disease.

Shunt procedures are the most numerous operations performed by neurosurgeons today, and surgeons insert these devices in the belief that the success of their surgical wizardry validates Dandy's dictum that water flows from the inside of the brain to the outside. But do these successful operations prove Dandy to be right?

Carbon dioxide, a gas, comes out of the hollow lungs, but it is not produced there; it comes from cells all over the body. No physician would assign carbon dioxide production to the lungs simply because an endotracheal tube allows carbon dioxide to leave the lungs.

Urine comes out of the hollow bladder, but it is not produced there; it comes from the kidneys some distance away. No physician would assign urine production to the bladder simply because a bladder catheter drains urine away.

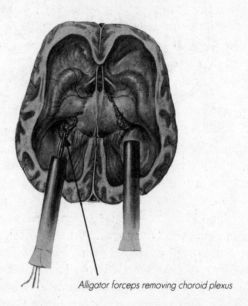

Alligator forceps removing choroid plexus

Fig. 13.5 For patients with meningitis who developed a 'blocked sub-arachnoid pathway', Dandy proposed the heroic but unsuccessful operation of choroid plexus removal, thinking wrongly that the flow of water into the ventricle would be reduced by this procedure

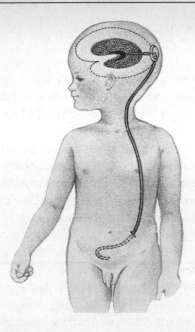

Fig. 13.6 Shunts are tunnelled under the skin to drain excess fluid from the brain to the abdomen

But physicians, chiefly neurosurgeons, drain spinal fluid from the hollow brain and jump to the conclusion that the fluid is produced in the ventricle by the choroid plexus, as Dandy taught.

If ventricular water moved in exactly the opposite direction, if the choroid plexus were the major pathway for water to leave the brain, not enter it, ventricle shunts would work just as effectively.

The success of ventricular shunting in hydrocephalus has led my busy colleagues, neurosurgeons, to believe in Dandy's paradigm as a fundamental fact of physiology, as have physicians and scientists of all kinds. Who, after all, knew the most about the hollow brain? Without doubt, the neurosurgeons.

Dandy's experiments were done in the fast lane of science, the Hunterian laboratory of Johns Hopkins. Only three years before, the Flexner report had championed the scientific, laboratory-based medicine that was practised at Johns Hopkins as the model that all other medical schools should copy. It was that report that triggered the decision of the Harvard Medical School to construct the Peter Bent Brigham Hospital and to recruit Cushing to run it. The Hunterian laboratory had seen the revolutionary pituitary experiments of Cushing; indeed, Dandy had been there to see some of them himself, and Dandy must have felt the pressure to produce that permeates the competitive institutions that wish to stay not only in the fast lane but also at the head of the pack.

Dandy's experiments were performed with no control animals, with no record of the number of animals operated on, with no regard for inter-species variability, with no record of the time base, with no histological correlation, with no attempt to quantify the differences and with no involvement of a neutral scientist. He did them essentially alone without any experienced scientific colleagues; William Blackfan, who joined him, was equally inexperienced. But the lack of controls, the absence of numbers, the disregard for brain chemistry, the belief that brain tissue was as inert as a rubber balloon, the narrowness of the interpretation of data, the quick transference of the laboratory results to the operating room and the refusal to acknowledge that the operations didn't work are the most distressing features.

One of Dandy's experiments, cursorily described a few pages ago, reveals how wrong his investigations were. Surgeons who have lived in the days of the 'iodine prep', a method of skin cleansing that was employed decades ago to sterilize surgical fields, repeatedly witnessed severe burns of the back from excessive iodine applied in a sloppy way to the abdomen. Some of these burns resulted in a full thickness skin loss. This substance would be the last thing on the lab shelf that an experienced surgeon would put in the brain. A destructive chemical 'burn' of the brain's cortex many inches away would be assured by the migration of the iodine. Dandy, with no surgical experience to guide him, employed iodine to make a 'scar' around the mid brain, but the experienced eye sees in his own photographs the telltale signs of cortical destruction; the enlarged ventricles he described as 'hydrocephalus' are impossible to distinguish from the brain atrophy that attends nerve cell destruction. Dandy performed this experiment on one animal, yet it became a keystone to his argument. What is more remarkable is the uncritical acclaim this experiment received.

Dandy was so convinced that his 1911 experiments had yielded the 'truth' that he ceased asking questions about the hollow brain and vacated the experimental animal laboratory.

Flushed by his laboratory successes and the acclaim they had received, Dandy injected air into the ventricles of humans; air did not pass into the brain but remained in the ventricles. This supported his notion that brain tissue was inert and would behave exactly as a rubber balloon. Moreover, air could be manipulated over the outside of the brain along the pathway for water that he thought he had demonstrated there. These splendid pictures cemented Dandy's paradigm in the minds of brain scientists far more than his animal studies had done. The radiology suite became the experimental laboratory for brain water, and thousands of human X-rays seemed to prove Dandy to be correct. Now it is clear that air injected into the brain does not behave at all like brain water; it follows very different pathways.

Almost as soon as they were performed, Dandy's experiments were heralded all over the world. Hopkins, and neurosurgery, had done it again. As Cushing had discovered the *raison d'être* for the pituitary in that institution, his successor, Dandy, had discovered the *raison d'être* for the hollow ventricles of the brain. The world accepted that Dandy found the 'truth' about the pathway that water took through the brain. He was joined by a broad group of supporters from both science and medicine to claim that he had made sense of ventricular anatomy, described the physiology of the ventricular system, explained ventricular pathology, that is, hydrocephalus, developed diagnostic tests for ventricular disease and designed and performed cures for ventricular diseases.

Look carefully at that list. It includes everything that is pertinent to the hollow brain: the anatomy, the physiology, the pathology, the diagnosis and the cure.

Dandy's paradigm was much like Galen's. He skewered many different facets of the ventricle to form a paradigm that almost defied attack. He had covered every base. Moreover, as Galen had built his paradigm on Aristotle's holy pneuma, Dandy built his paradigm on the holiest concept in medicine – circulation. His third circulation of brain water gained attention and respect because it so closely resembled the first circulation of Harvey (blood) and the second circulation of Hunter (lymph).

My criticisms are these.

First, neither choroid plexectomy nor third ventriculostomy is effective therapy for hydrocephalus. If Dandy's paradigm were correct, these operations would be effective.

Second, there is solid evidence that the choroid plexus absorbs water; the amount of water that it secretes and the amount of water it absorbs are difficult to determine. There are regional differences in the lining of the ventricle and also in the function of the choroid plexus and it is quite possible that the choroid may handle water like the kidney does; it may release water in one place and absorb it in another.

Third, the ventricles are not the impermeable rubber balloons that Dandy assumed. Although air may not pass into the brain, water in the ventricle certainly does. Much larger molecules, such as horseradish peroxidase, 20,000 times larger than the size of a water molecule, readily pass from the ventricle into the brain itself.

Fourth, if special 'fishing nets' are cast into the waters of the ventricle, at least 317 separate kinds of peptides can be recovered. The 'net' that does this is a simple test: two-dimensional gel electrophoresis. Such gels move molecules at different rates because of electrical charges and molecular weights. One tiny drop of ventricular fluid would produce 317 different spots on such a gel. Yet if this same net is cast outside the brain, just at the outlet of the ventricular system, there are only 309 different spots. The lack of an increase in these spots at the outlet of the ventricle damns the Dandy paradigm. The accumulation of more peptides in the ventricle suggests that water may be moving in a direction precisely opposite to that preached by Dandy: towards the choroid plexus. The 'sewer-like' function that Dandy ascribed to the ventricles cannot be supported by these two-dimensional gel data (see Fig. 13.7).

Fifth, if synthetic brain hormones that have a powerful effect on the endocrine glands of the body are placed in the ventricle, they

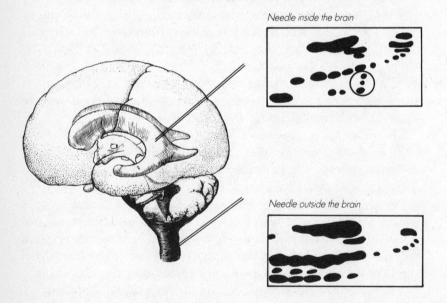

Needle inside the brain

Needle outside the brain

Fig. 13.7 Circled dots are evidence that some proteins do not leave the ventricles

may have no effect whatsoever on these glands. By Dandy's paradigm, these substances should be washed out of the brain and into the bloodstream where they could exert their action.

Sixth, if the powerful hormone vasopressin, or ADH, is injected into the blood, the body will retain water. If ADH is injected into the ventricle the opposite happens: the body loses water. This demonstrates that this substance does not leave the brain along Dandy's time-honoured pathway. For whatever reason, the brain 'traps' ADH in the ventricle or, possibly, there is a current of water that flows towards the choroid plexus.

Seventh, in an earlier day when the hazards of radioisotopes were not so well known, radioactive substances were put in the ventricles of humans. The isotopes appeared in the blood almost instantly, within the first minute, but did not appear outside the ventricle until much later, proof that they had not travelled to the bloodstream along Dandy's pathway.

These are only seven observations that do not fit with Dandy's notions on brain water; there are many more.

Dandy's paradigm is a mismeme that ranks with that of Aristotle's hollow, pneuma-filled arteries and Galen's four humours. If the evidence against Dandy is so certain, why is his paradigm still included in the leading journals as a basic 'truth'? Why is it still accepted by the best educated psychiatrists, neurologists and neurosurgeons and the brightest neuroanatomists, neurophysiologists and neurochemists?

First and foremost, nearly all of these groups are content with Dandy's answer to the question, 'Why is the brain hollow?' For their own reasons, they see no substance in the question – nowhere that its answer could lead. Neurosurgeons, watching every day the success of shunts based upon Dandy's paradigm, see no reason to ask the question. The intellectual security that neurosurgeons gained from the Dandy paradigm not only for their hydrocephalus operations but also for most of their intracranial procedures is well known. Although Dandy's explanation may be wrong, they base much of what they do on the simple thesis that big ventricles are unhealthy; shunts, and ventricular drains, yield smaller ventricles and healthier patients. Their functioning shunts could mean that brain water leaves the brain through the choroid plexus; for the diseases neurosurgeons deal with it makes no difference, the paradigm works. The acceptance of the Dandy paradigm makes it easier for everyone to work with the paradigm of the electrically driven brain.

Most scientists today are reductionists. To challenge Dandy's paradigm requires a holistic approach to the brain. Those at the top in brain science gained their pedestals by knowing more and more about less and less. To challenge the Dandy paradigm requires a knowledge of brain anatomy, physiology, pathology, radiology and surgery. Very few of today's scientists would claim to have a sound grasp of each of these disciplines.

Information overload is a major contributor to the longevity of Dandy's mismeme. Dandy's paradigm has been quoted by so many scientific authors in so many different ways and for so many different reasons that it runs like a golden thread from publication to publication. In a tug-of-war between one new reference and a million old references, the battle would resemble an ant trying to outpull an elephant.

Many decades ago, Cushing raised serious questions about Dandy's paradigm. Tom Milhorat, a neurosurgeon in New York, raised similar questions in a well-reasoned article written in 1975. Those criticisms were published when the paradigm of an electrically driven brain was in vogue and there was no urgency to confront the many obvious inconsistencies in the Dandy paradigm. But if one accepts the notion that the brain is a hormonally modulated gland, then the question, 'Why is the brain hollow?', looms as central.

Billions of dollars have been spent to take photographs of distant planets, to pilfer a few stones from the gullies of the moon and to scratch a remote-controlled shovel into the surface of Mars to see if it contained life. While this fantastic effort to understand more about the surfaces of distant planets has been going on, the inside surface of the human brain has remained largely unexplored. The photographic exploration of its inner surface has been much more haphazard than that of the planets, few molecules have been pilfered from between the cilia of the ventricle and no remote-control shovels have been sent into the brain to tell us more about life on the surface of the ventricle.

The ventricles of the brain are much more than fluid-filled cushions that make your somersaults and football games go better. Although these spaces appear at first glance to be the cleanest spaces in the body, they contain a treasury of endocrine information about the brain that is unattainable anywhere else. It seems certain that only by tapping into this treasury of hormones will the mysteries of the hollow brain gland be revealed.

More and more evidence suggests that the brain was given its hollow form to fulfil endocrine functions. The human ventricle is the best place, perhaps the only reliable place, to search for correlations between human behaviour and brain hormones.

Dandy, without doubt, achieved greatness. He boldly charged into the no-man's land of the brain's ventricle, both in the operating room and in the laboratory, and showed to the world that it was a space that surgeons could enter. He did for the inside of mankind's microcosm what Neil Armstrong did for mankind's macrocosm. He was also a teacher of high standards, a compassionate physician, an inventive surgeon, and a good writer; to this day his book *The Brain* is the best single volume in the field of neurosurgery.

Like many young academic physicians before and after him, Dandy was asked by his institution to do research to obtain new information about the mysteries of the body. But Dandy, like many before and after him, was also asked to care for the sick, to be involved with their anxieties and their diseases, to care and, sometimes, to cure.

He fell into the trap that befalls most young people who are asked to partake of this schizophrenia: he spoke as a research scientist to his fellow physicians. But when asked to address scientists, he spoke of disease like a pastor.

Modern brain scientists use Dandy's mismeme to protect their belief that electricity is the stuff of thought; it combines ventricular anatomy, physiology, pathology, diagnosis and therapy in a strong paradigm, which virtually defies attack. As long as it is in place, physiologists do not need to explore the 'wetness' of the brain.

Shoreline of Wonder

The question, 'Why is the brain hollow?', may be the most important unanswered question about the brain. Since the human brain has been the shaping force of our civilization, this question might be regarded as one of the most important biological questions of our times.

Why is this question so important?

Look back at the age of Galen. The hollowness of the heart had been established by other anatomists; Galen had assigned functions to each of its chambers. The right heart allowed the liver to pump blood through it into veins; the left heart allowed the to-and-fro movement of pneuma and sanquine. Galen even fabricated a hollowness that wasn't there. He placed hollow pores in the heart's septum that allowed 'sooty stuff' to move from the venous blood into the arterial blood.

As long as Galen's errors about the heart remained unquestioned, all other portions of his philosophy could remain in place. Vesalius first questioned the existence of Galen's hollow pores in the septum. Later William Harvey asked the question, 'Why is the heart hollow?', and together these questions destroyed the grip that Galen's nonsenses had held in people's minds.

Few would have predicted that the discovery of the circulation of blood would have changed the way philosophers view the world, theologians conceive of God, or astronomers look at the stars, yet all of that happened. In retrospect the question, 'Why is the heart hollow?', changed the course of civilization as much as any other single question. If the question, 'Why is the heart hollow?', had a profound impact on all intellectual disciplines, would you expect any less of the question, 'Why is the brain hollow?'

14

Issues For Those Who Are Well

*P*lato, committed to the perfection of the sphere, postulated a
soul-force that came from a spherical universe into the
spherical cranium. Aristotle, led astray by air-filled arteries,
concluded that heaven-sent pneuma empowered a rational
soul residing in the heart. Galen's belief in humours led him to
think the soul-force – animal spirit – was stored in the ventricles.
Descartes was more specific: he concluded that the pineal gland
was the seat of the soul. The group-thinkers who followed Galvani
have placed the soul in the left brain and made brain electricity its
helmsman. In the past decade, as regulating hormones have been
found throughout the body, the soul has lost its home. It is scattered everywhere – in the brain, the gut, the ovary, the pituitary
and the adrenal; if paracrinologists are correct, every cell contains
the well-chiselled molecules that give life to the soul and guidance
to the mind.

Three laboratory techniques – electronmicroscopy, immunohistochemistry and hybridization histochemistry – have allowed
scientists to peek into cells to see this new soul and mind essence
(see Fig. 14.1).

When the soul was in the spherical head, the hollow heart, the
ventricles, the pineal, or the left brain, philosophers and scientists
who were interested in such things could keep one force – one
'reduction' – central to their thoughts. Modern thinkers about the
soul must contemplate a plethora of regulating hormones, each
with a long Latin name. Table 14.1 illustrates the abbreviations
that can more easily describe the numerous, ubiquitous guiding
forces that whirl about inside the body.

Most, if not all, of these substances are not found only in the
brain. They are produced in many remote glands and organs. Table
14.2 shows their sites of production outside the brain.

Table 14.1   BRAIN HORMONES

Regulatory Hormone	Abbreviation
Acetylcholine	ACh
Adrenalin	EPI
Norepinephrine	NE
Serotonin	5-HT
Histamine	H
Dopamine	DA
Gamma aminobutyrate	GABA
Glutamate	GLU
Glycine	GLY
Melatonin	MEL
Muscarinic Nuerophysin	NP (Mus)
Nicotinic Neurophysin	NP (Nic)
Arginine Vasopressin	AVP
Lysine Vasopressin	LVP
Angiotensin	A2
Thyroid Hormone	TH
Thyroid Releasing Hormone	TRH
Luteinizing Hormone	LH
Gonadotropin Releasing Hormone	GNRH
Growth Hormone	GH
Growth Hormone Releasing Hormone	GHRH
Somatostatin	SRIF
Corticotropin Releasing Hormone	CRH
Prolactin	PRL
Substance P	SUB-P
Neurotensin	NTSN
Vasoactive Intestinal Peptide	VIP
Gastrin	GAST
Cholecystokinen	CCK
Bombesin	BOMB
Adrenocorticotropin	ACTH
Pro-opiomelanocortin	31-K
Lipotropin	LPH
Endorphin	ENDO
Dynorphin	DYN
Enkephalin	ENK
Melanotropin Stimulating Hormone	MSH
Insulin	INS

Table 14.2 SITES OF HORMONE PRODUCTION OUTSIDE THE BRAIN

Regulatory Hormone	Other Organ Sites				
	Brain	Pituitary	Adrenal	Gut	Gonads
Acetylcholine	●	●	●	●	●
Adrenalin	●	●	●	●	●
Noradrenalin	●	●	●	●	●
Serotonin	●	●	●	●	●
Histamine	●	●	●	●	●
Dopamine	●	●	●	●	●
GABA	●	●	●	●	●
Glutamate	●	●	●	●	●
Glycine	●	●	●	●	●
Melatonin	●				
Muscarinic NP	●	●			
Nicotinic NP	●	●			
AVP	●	●		●	●
LVP	●	●		●	●
Angiotensin	●	●			
Thyroid Hormone	●	●			
TRH	●	●			
LH	●	●			
GNRH	●	●			
Growth Hormone	●	●			
GHRH	●	●			
SRIF	●	●			
CRH	●	●		●	
Prolactin	●	●			
Substance P	●	●		●	
Neurotensin	●	●		●	
VIP	●	●		●	
Gastrin	●	●		●	
Cholecystokinen	●	●		●	
Bombesin	●	●		●	
ACTH	●	●		●	
31-K	●	●	●	●	●
Lipotropin	●	●	●	●	●
Endorphin	●	●	●	●	●
Dynorphin	●	●	●	●	●
Enkephalin	●	●	●	●	●
MSH	●	●	●	●	●
Insulin	●		●		

Table 14.3 shows the kinds of behaviour that are modified by regulatory brain hormones. None of the hormones is linked specifically to a behaviour in this table, but it emphasizes the opportunity for correlating certain kinds of behaviour with certain hormones.

Table 14.3   REGULATORY HORMONES AND BEHAVIOUR

Regulatory Hormone	Behaviour
Acetylcholine	Memory
Adrenalin	
Noradrenalin	
Serotonin	Joy
GABA	
Dopamine	Thirst
Muscurinic Neurophysin	
Nicotinic Neurophysin	Hunger
Vasopressin	
Angiotensin	Satiation
Thyroid Hormone	
Thyroid Releasing Hormone	Orgasm
Luteinizing Hormone	
Gonadotropin Releasing Hormone	Sleep
Growth Hormone	
Somatostatin	Addiction
Corticotropin Releasing Hormone	
Prolactin	Opiate overdose
Substance P	
Neurotensin	Sorrow
Vasoactive Intestinal Peptide	
Gastrin	Rage
Cholecystokinen	
Bombesin	Depression
ACTH	
Pro-opiomelanocortin	Suicide
Lipotropin	
Endorphin	Fear
Dynorphin	
Enkephalin	Peace
Melanotropin Stimulating Hormone	
Insulin	Pain

Table 14.4 lists the many different bodily functions that are influenced by regulatory hormones. In this table, specific correlations are not made, but the need for such connections is apparent.

Table 14.4   BODILY FUNCTIONS INFLUENCED BY REGULATORY HORMONES

Regulatory Hormone	Body Function
Acetylcholine	Sleep
Adrenalin	
Noradrenalin	
Serotonin	Pain
GABA	
Dopamine	Blood pressure
Muscarinic Neurophysin	
Nicotinic Neurophysin	Digestion
Vasopressin	
Angiotensin	Blood coagulation
Thyroid Hormone	
Thyroid Releasing Hormone	Immunity
Luteinizing Hormone	
Gonadotropin Releasing Hormone	Sexual function
Growth Hormone	
Somatostatin	Reproduction
Corticotropin Releasing Hormone	
Prolactin	Temperature control
Substance P	
Neurotensin	Bowel motility
Vasoactive Intestinal Peptide	
Gastrin	Gastric acidity
Cholecystokinen	
Bombesin	Skin rashes
ACTH	
Pro-opiomelanocortin	Asthma
Lipotropin	
Endorphin	Ageing
Dynorphin	
Enkephalin	Obesity
Melanotropin Stimulating Hormone	
Insulin	Arthritic stiffness

To demonstrate correlations, lines must be drawn between the different hormones and the different brain behaviours or body functions. Table 14.5 shows how one hormone, vasopressin, might influence several different kinds of behaviour.

Table 14.5 CORRELATIONS BETWEEN VASOPRESSIN AND BEHAVIOUR

Adrenalin	Memory
Acetylcholine	Memory
Adrenalin	
Noradrenalin	
Serotonin	Joy
GABA	
Dopamine	Thirst
Muscarinic Neurophysin	
Nicotinic Neurophysin	Hunger
Vasopressin	
Angiotensin	Satiation
Thyroid Hormone	
Thyroid Releasing Hormone	Orgasm
Luteinizing Hormone	
Gonadotropin Releasing Hormone	Sleep
Growth Hormone	
Somatostatin	Addiction
Corticotropin Releasing Hormone	
Prolactin	Opiate overdose
Substance P	
Neurotensin	Sorrow
Vasoactive Intestinal Peptide	
Gastrin	Rage
Cholecystokinen	
Bombesin	Depression
ACTH	
Pro-opiomelanocortin	Suicide
Lipotropin	
Endorphin	Fear
Dynorphin	
Enkephalin	Peace
Melanotropin Stimulating Hormone	
Insulin	Pain

Conversely, Table 14.6 shows the possible hormonal correlations for 'pain'.

Table 14.6 CORRELATIONS BETWEEN PAIN AND SEVERAL HORMONES

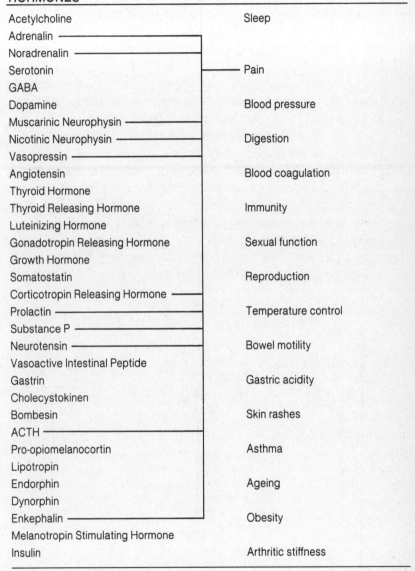

Acetylcholine	Sleep
Adrenalin	
Noradrenalin	
Serotonin	Pain
GABA	
Dopamine	Blood pressure
Muscarinic Neurophysin	
Nicotinic Neurophysin	Digestion
Vasopressin	
Angiotensin	Blood coagulation
Thyroid Hormone	
Thyroid Releasing Hormone	Immunity
Luteinizing Hormone	
Gonadotropin Releasing Hormone	Sexual function
Growth Hormone	
Somatostatin	Reproduction
Corticotropin Releasing Hormone	
Prolactin	Temperature control
Substance P	
Neurotensin	Bowel motility
Vasoactive Intestinal Peptide	
Gastrin	Gastric acidity
Cholecystokinen	
Bombesin	Skin rashes
ACTH	
Pro-opiomelanocortin	Asthma
Lipotropin	
Endorphin	Ageing
Dynorphin	
Enkephalin	Obesity
Melanotropin Stimulating Hormone	
Insulin	Arthritic stiffness

From these tables, you would quickly decide that one kind of behaviour or one illness may be linked to more than one hormone and that a single brain hormone may be associated with more than one regulating function.

No scientist knows just now how many regulatory hormones there are. But the question is clear: does the body employ individual hormones like the letters of an alphabet?

If it does, scientists may not find thousands of individual hormones; the list may be much shorter. But the number of regulatory hormones in its 'alphabet' is very important. If the mind employs individual brain hormones as letters of an endocrine alphabet, one extra brain hormone would confuse every kind of regulating signal.

But even before the size and form of the brain's hormonal alphabet is determined, correlations are possible between certain hormones and certain body and brain activities.

There are several hormones that are important to memory, one of the mind's most important functions. Vasopressin, ACTH and MSH have all been implicated in learning in animal experiments. If these hormones are important to normal memory processes, might they not be important to disorders of memory? There is a silent epidemic of senile dementia in the world. If these hormones are as important to humans as they are to animal learning, it is possible that the same hormones could be important to senile dementia, indeed to all other diseases that cause memory loss. The question

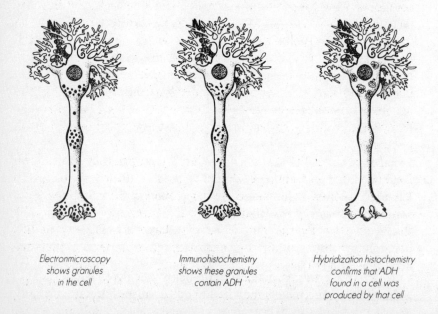

Electronmicroscopy
shows granules
in the cell

Immunohistochemistry
shows these granules
contain ADH

Hybridization histochemistry
confirms that ADH
found in a cell was
produced by that cell

Fig. 14.1 In the study of an ADH-producing cell, different techniques show different things

immediately arises, 'Could hormones be given to patients with memory problems, just as insulin is given to patients with diabetes?'

Norman Cousins, in his book, *The Anatomy of an Illness*, sets out his experience with the healing power of joy. His severe bone and joint problems were driven from his body by belly laughter triggered by viewing old comic movies. Cousins postulated that 'hormones of happiness' are released when the dog wags his tail or when people are extremely happy. He found healing in happiness and proclaims in a compelling way that such hormones must exist. But the existence of these hormones in the blood of either animals or people is almost impossible for scientists to discern; the very act of blood removal creates stress and unhappiness. One of the best pieces of scientific evidence to support Cousins's notion that there is a chemistry of 'joy' and 'sorrow' can be found in the chemical analysis of tears. In anyone, a stroke of good fortune can trigger the release of 'happy' tears; these have a very different molecular make-up from 'sad' tears. The analysis of tears confirms that the body has one chemistry for joy and another for sadness.

Thirst is by far the easiest behaviour to measure quantitatively in animal experiments, and more is known about it than any other kind of behaviour. It is modified by regulatory hormones, much like memory and joy. 'Angiotensin' is the hormone most involved in the control of water appetite; in animals a small amount of it injected into the blood vessels going to the brain causes a powerful desire to drink. It is in the area of salt and water appetite that the importance of brain hormones has become most obvious. Since hypertension is so obviously related to salt and water balance, many scientists are devoting themselves to the study of the hormones that control salt and water appetite, believing that new knowledge in this area will bring with it the control of high blood pressure.

Hunger, like thirst, is controlled by regulatory hormones. Experiments in animals have linked caloric appetite to 'cholecystokinen', a hormone that was found in the intestines. Now some scientists suggest that more of this hormone is produced by the brain than by the gut. Mice that have a deficiency of this hormone in their brain, for example, have appetites that are insatiable. They will eat virtually anything in sight, including their cage. Conversely, sheep who have been given this hormone into their brain refuse to eat anything. Insulin, the hormone linked to diabetes, is even more strongly connected to food hunger. Many scientists predict that an understanding of brain hormones will allow the ultimate in diet control; a medication that takes away the appetite for food but does nothing else.

Satiation, like thirst and hunger, is a condition that is determined by hormones. Each kind of appetite has its own satiating substance, but most scientific interest has focused on the satiation of caloric appetite. Knowing about the hormonal control of satiation could lead to the development of other kinds of diet-control pills. The mysterious disease, anorexia nervosa, stemming from a feeling of continual satiation, has been linked both to bombesin and vasopressin. New knowledge about the endrocrinology of this common, dreaded disease of young women seems to offer the only hope for its therapy.

Sexual orgasm is at once mysterious and poorly understood, but most scientists believe it begins and ends in the brain, not the pelvis. The appetite for orgasm drives both male and female scientists at night, but oddly, in their daytime lives, they find very little time to study it. Many have suggested that the opiate-like hormones endorphin and enkephalin are responsible for sexual pleasure, but the evidence to support that is anything but certain. In many animals these hormones will trigger contractions in the vas deferens – the tiny tube that carries sperm – and this may be the best reason to link these hormones to orgasm. One new brain hormone, 'gonadotropin releasing hormone', may play a key role in male erections, giving hope to those with impotence.

Sleep has been very closely linked to brain hormones. Harvard scientists have isolated a substance in the ventricular fluid of a sleeping goat that will cause another goat to drift off to sleep. Sleep may be the most mysterious thing that the brain does: nobody yet knows why we get tired, why we sleep, and what benefit sleep brings our bodies. Yet nearly all of the body's endocrine rhythms are correlated to sleep, and some of the most mysterious aspects of sleep, such as rapid eye movement sleep, are directly linked to surges in brain hormones in the blood. Knowing why goats sleep, or why humans do or do not sleep would help society immensely, for insomnia is one of the most common complaints that patients relate to their physicians.

Addiction to opiate drugs of any kind – heroin is one kind of opiate – is governed by the interactions of hormones and hormone receptors in the brain. Nature has given the brain the capacity to produce its own opiate-like drugs and has also provided the brain with opiate receptors on many kinds of brain cells. Nature has established this system so that the brain can treat itself during emergencies. One of the explanations for drug addiction rests in the belief that injections of external opiates turn off the brain machinery for the production of internal opiates. Each brain cell that normally produces an internal opiate – endorphin, enkephalin, or dynorphin – is turned off, sensing that enough brain opiates are already present. The force that comes into an addict's life results from a shut-down of the brain's ability to produce brain opiates; as long as addicts continue to receive external opium such as heroin addiction will remain. Addiction ceases when the brain resumes the production of its own opiate-like hormones.

Rage in animals has been linked to the release of catecholamines. Many scientists believe that at the moment of extreme rage the brain is filled with catecholamines – either adrenalin, noradrenalin, or serotonin. These in turn may trigger the release of many other hormones, each of which could affect behaviour and cloud judgement. Knowing about the regulatory hormones responsible for aggressive behaviour might reduce the numbers in our nation's jails.

Depression, especially the kind of depression which is always 'down' and never 'up', 'unipolar depression', creates immense changes in the endocrine system. These alterations are especially evident in the brain/pituitary/adrenal axis and most easily assessed by measuring the amount of adrenal hormone, 'cortisol', that is in the bloodstream. Typically, those with this kind of depression have blood levels of cortisol that are far too high and without the typical diurnal variation. Such depressed patients do not suppress their secretion of cortisol when given a synthetic hormone called 'decadron', an indication that the brain has decided to increase the output of hormones from the pituitary and the adrenal. Why this should be is not certain, but it suggests that the brain may be deficient in these hormones or other hormones and directs distant glands to secrete more of them to treat the deficiency.

The chemical analysis of the brains of suicide victims shows special kinds of hormone profiles, very different from normal brains, indicating that these people, who are obviously depressed, have endocrine abnormalities in their brains.

Fear, like rage, releases 'catecholamines'. But judging from many different kinds of animal experiments, many other hormones are also released, including vasopressin, endorphin and prolactin. Many of these hormones are gut hormones that increase gastric and intestinal motility, making it common for bowel incontinence to develop as a result of fear.

For centuries, Vedic priests have maintained that meditation is the path to peace, that there are substances in the body that can be released by an effort of the mind that fill the mind with peace. Many Western scientists now acknowledge that some such peace-giving hormones are released during meditation. What they are is uncertain, but there can be no doubt that many endocrine relationships are changed.

Pain perception is modified by many hormones besides the opiate hormones; scientists now acknowledge that the greatest hope for the understanding and treatment of pain lies in deciphering the complex endocrine relationships that are triggered by pain; the list of hormones involved in pain modulation grows longer and now includes endorphin, enkephalin, dynorphin and substance P. The stimulus of pain releases these substances, which form links with the hormone receptors in brain cells. Nature has stored these hormones in the brain for the treatment of pain.

The correlation between individual brain hormones and different kinds of brain and body activities has raised the expectations of brain scientists. They anticipate the day when brain illnesses in humans can be treated with hormones. It would be easier for these scientists if all animals spoke the same endocrine language, for then correlations made in the laboratory could be quickly moved to the bedside. Unfortunately such is not the case. The hormone prolactin, for example, has at least seventy-eight different functions in seventy-eight different species. Just as the same vowel-sounds and consonants are used differently by different peoples, hormones are used by different species to convey different messages. This forces scientists to establish functional correlations in the species of their concern.

Some observations in animal experiments may point the way, but ultimately correlations that will benefit mankind must be established in human studies.

One problem that stymies the development of endocrine neurology is the 'blood-brain barrier'. To understand this vexing problem, we need to look more closely at the differences between neuroendocrinology and endocrine neurology.

Neuroendocrinology, or brain-to-gland relationships, involves a pyramidal hierarchy of glands with the brain at the top. The controlling messages from the brain are amplified as they move down this pyramid; that is, as the hormonal messages move like falling dominoes, each message lasts longer, travels further and affects greater numbers of other organs. Many have referred to this process as 'cascading hormonal amplification' or 'hormonal amplification'.

All endocrine glands except the testes and the brain have perme-

able capillaries – blood vessels are poked full of holes exactly as
Galen described (see Fig. 14.2). It is the presence of such capillary
pores that allows the process of hormonal amplification. Hormones
formed by cells in glands first leak into the bloodstream through
these holes, then flow through the bloodstream to leak out of it in
some other gland.

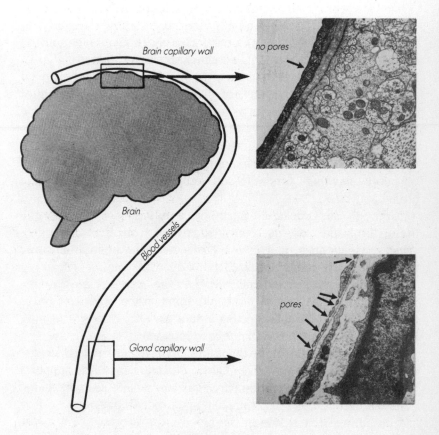

Fig. 14.2 The electronmicrograph of a capillary of a gland shows the many 'pores' through which
hormones flow in and out of the gland. Capillaries in the brain do not have such pores

As hormones are carried from gland to gland by the bloodstream, excessive or diminished levels of circulating hormones can
be established with relative ease. By blood samples, the 'signals'
passing from one gland to another can be intercepted. If a deficiency is found, replacement therapy can be given with the knowledge that the leaky capillaries will allow it to reach its target.

The brain has all the characteristics of a gland except one –

leaky capillaries – and the sturdy brain capillaries are collectively called the 'blood-brain barrier'. This barrier can be easily demonstrated by injecting a blue dye into an animal; every other organ (except the testicle) turns blue, but the blood-brain barrier keeps the brain as white as snow.

Although all the hormones in the endocrine system are carried by the bloodstream to the brain, the presence of the blood-brain barrier prevents most hormones from penetrating it.

A mechanism that might be described as 'hormonal deamplification' limits the effect that the endocrine system can have on the nervous system. As hormonal amplification is the hallmark of all of the brain-to-gland relationships of neuroendocrinology, hormonal deamplification is the hallmark of all gland-to-brain relationships of endocrine neurology. This is a fundamental difference between the two sciences.

Some kinds of hormones, the 'steroids', pass readily into the brain, but the 'peptide' hormones produced by the pituitary, the gut, and any other glands do not easily pass through the wall of brain capillaries.

Although the process of hormonal amplification begins in the brain, the brain remains silently separated from the noisy endocrine consequences. It does not easily hear the endocrine music produced by the other glands of the body.

Is the brain really hormonally deaf? As the brain's prime function is to receive, store and sort through information of all kinds, it is untenable to believe that it doesn't want to hear or doesn't need to hear the endocrine music that it orchestrates.

Since the discovery of the blood-brain barrier seventy years ago, it has been assigned a passive quality. But more evidence supports the view that the blood-brain barrier is active, like a sophisticated machine that pumps some things in and other things out.

The pumps that reside in the blood-brain barrier are not well understood, but for one hormone, insulin, pumps have been found that suggest that the passage of hormones into the brain is determined by a dynamic process. The pumps in the blood-brain barrier may allow the brain to pick and choose from the vast number of hormones that are continually flowing through it. As more is learned about these pumps, the endocrine silence of the brain looks increasingly like an active process and one that is as finely tuned as the more easily studied process of cascading hormonal amplification.

The brain is not hormonally deaf. If the blood-brain barrier is selectively opened and closed, if hormonal deamplification is as active as hormonal amplification, a vast new area of science and medicine unfolds. Many poorly understood aspects of normal behaviour might be explained by a dynamically changing blood-brain barrier. Orgasm, for example, may result from the transient opening of the brain's capillaries; blood-borne 'hormones of happiness' may be allowed into the brain during the brief interval that the brain's capillaries become permeable. Many behavioural diseases may result from a mistuned blood-brain barrier that allows the brain to receive too few or too many hormones. Depression, for example, may result from capillaries that are too tight and do not allow the 'hormones of happiness' into the brain. The understanding of the fine-tuning of the blood-brain barrier would help physicians to understand diseases and allow them to develop new kinds of routes by which hormones could be fed to the brain.

Although a dynamic, finely tuned blood-brain barrier seems likely, there can be no escape from this reality: the measurement of hormones in the bloodstream of patients will not reflect the endocrine activity in the brain. It is this impasse that forces me to believe that catheters must be placed into the cerebral ventricles if the major diseases of the mind are to be understood.

Suppose that a brain scientist, convinced that he or she knows which hormones are responsible for 'closing gates' in animals, wants to confirm this in humans. Where should the sampling needle be placed? The blood-brain barrier makes it unlikely that meaningful hormonal/behavioural correlations can be established by blood measurements alone. Neither excessive levels nor diminished levels of brain hormones would be reflected in circulating blood. As certainly as the process of 'hormonal deamplification' limits the flow of body hormones into the brain, the same process limits the flow from the brain to the body.

Correlations between brain hormones and behaviour obtained by brain biopsies are ethically and morally impossible, even though the measurement of brain hormones in brain tissue affords the best opportunity for such correlations.

Many scientists, intent on making correlations between behaviour and brain hormones, especially abnormal behaviour and brain hormones, have turned to the lumbar spinal fluid for analysis. The spinal cord does not extend to the end of the spinal canal in humans, leaving a large fluid-filled space that can be quite easily tapped with a delicate needle in a relatively easy and safe procedure. Lamentably, data from the two-dimensional gel studies demonstrate that the greatest array of brain hormones is found in the ventricle, not in the spinal fluid.

Of all of the possible sampling sites for brain hormones, ventricular fluid appears to be the best. If the brain is regarded as a gland, its hollowness must be given a new light. It is unlikely that the cerebral ventricles have been set in place solely for the production and transportation of brain water. The ventricles can be regarded as centrally placed ducts that contain hormones – the most brain hormones of any single sampling site. As in the hollow heart and the hollow stomach, catheters will be needed in the centre of the hollow brain if we expect to make valid correlations between brain hormones and behaviour.

Placing catheters in the ventricles of patients with hydrocephalus, tumours and head trauma is done frequently and with remarkable safety. The advent of the CAT and NMR scanners to guide catheters into the brain significantly reduces the risk of this procedure, and I predict that in decades to come ventricular catheterization performed to measure hormone concentrations will become as routine as the measurement of lumbar 'pressure' is today.

An understanding of the limitations of blood sampling and lumbar fluid sampling forces the conclusion that only by placing catheters in the cerebral ventricles can the significance of brain hormones be understood. Since few human illnesses of the brain occur in laboratory animals, studies of human ventricular hormones may be the *sine qua non* of the new science of endocrine neurology.

Because many hormones may be linked to one kind of behaviour, a correlation between brain hormones and any kind of hormonally dependent activity must entail the measurement of not one but several hormones. This amplifies the task considerably; a single sample of blood or brain fluid might require forty-five separate analytical tests.

But other problems exist. Only by timing the sampling of brain hormones precisely with the event causing pain, for example, could correlations be established that would help our understanding of it. Quite obviously, this immensely magnifies the task at hand for 'normal' behavioural correlations. During sexual orgasm, for example, such correlations would have to be timed with exquisite care, perhaps during an interval of a few seconds. Paradoxically, correlations of brain hormones to 'abnormal' behaviour might be more reliable and give scientists better information. One would expect steady, long-lasting abnormalities, for example, in the disease, senile dementia; samples could be obtained at any time.

Although I am an avowed holist, I am forced to concede that the major diseases of the brain and the importance of brain hormones to brain function will only be understood by a very focused, very reductionistic procedure: ventricular catheterization (see Fig. 14.3). Only by such manoeuvres will hormone-related brain illnesses be understood and conquered.

Knowing that the brain is a gland gives the physician many new therapeutic options. Hormonal diseases of the brain, like endocrine diseases of the body, may be broken down into diseases of excessive secretion – hypersecretion – and diseases of diminished secretion – hyposecretion. Physicians might then design therapies that will replenish a hormone-hungry brain and design other therapies to block the effect of a hormone excess. But whatever they do

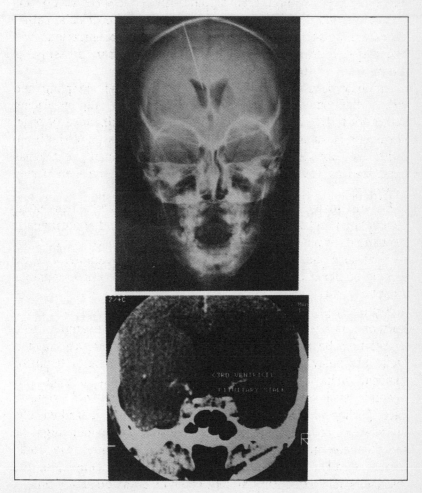

Fig. 14.3 New non-invasive CAT scans allow surgeons to see the ventricles

will depend on a precise measurement of brain hormones. It is with these therapeutic possibilities in mind that I advocate the measurement of ventricular hormones.

Table 14.7 lists the endocrine disorders of other glands. It is incomplete, but it does show that for each gland there are diseases of hyposecretion and hypersecretion. In every case where a hormone deficiency has been identified, substitution therapy of the appropriate hormone has led to cure. There is little doubt that similar 'magic' can be performed in the human brain.

Table 14.7   ENDOCRINE DISORDERS OF GLANDS

	Hypersecretion	Hyposecretion
Pituitary	Gigantism	Dwarfism
Thyroid	Graves Disease	Hypothyroidism
Adrenal	Cushing's Disease	Addison's Disease
Pancreas	Insulinoma	Diabetes
Parathyroids	Hypercalcemia	Hypocalcemia

Although I can only guess which brain diseases will stem from hyposecretion of brain hormones and which will stem from hypersecretion, one thing is clear at the outset. If diseases of hyposecretion can be identified, these diseases might be treated by hormonal replacement.

If deficiencies of brain hormones are established, when and where should the replacement be given? For any such therapy to be effective, the timing would have to be very precise. Again, diseases of chronic deficiency would be most easily managed. Senile dementia, for example, might be treated with a chronic infusion device.

The site of the therapy? Hormones given into the bloodstream would have no effect unless the blood-brain barrier could be opened in synchrony. Hormones given into the lumbar sack predictably would not make their way into the brain. As the hollowness of the brain dictates ventricular catheters for diagnosis, the ventricles appear to be the only feasible site for hormone replacement.

In 1927 most of the world thought the heart was an electrical organ; the electrocardiogram had confirmed it. A few brave physicians recognized that the electrical studies of the heart would lead down a dead-end street and attacked the central question of the hollow heart. The German physician who first placed a catheter in the hollow heart was thought to be mentally unbalanced. The physician, Dr Forssmann, performed that feat by himself and on himself. Although he was removed from his clinical responsibilities for his 'mental derangement', in 1955 the world cheered as he was awarded the Nobel Prize.

It was the surgical attack on the hollow heart – abhorrent, indeed 'crazy', to most – which led to the spectacular successes of modern cardiology.

Doubtless, physicians were slow to place catheters in the heart because they, like their patients, carried a primeval respect for it. To catheterize the heart was a desecration of something holy. As the mystique has gone from the heart, its problems have become much more tractable.

There is also little to fear in exploring the ventricles of the human brain. They are filled with hormones, and until the hormones swimming in these oceans are dredged out, countless millions of our fellows will remain with brain illnesses that can be neither understood nor treated. Many of their hormone-hungry brains may be fixed as easily as hormone-hungry bodies are fixed with thyroid hormone, insulin, oestrogen and testosterone, but that work cannot begin until cause and effect relationships between brain hormones and brain diseases have been established.

The next step in the effort to understand the human mind must be hormone analysis in the hollow brain glands of humans.

It is increasingly certain that the two brains, the right and left, are structurally and chemically different. Modern day CAT scans have confirmed this in humans, and endocrine studies of the left and right brain have confirmed this in animals.

It is also certain that people who have 'different' cerebral asymmetries – left handers – have 'different' bodies. Surprising structural differences in the brains of left handers and unsuspected differences in the bodies of left handers have been confirmed by

Norman Geschwind, the world's leading authority on the asymmetrical structure and function of the human brain. Countless times Geschwind has demonstrated both the advantages and the disadvantages of being a 'lefty'. The changes that he has found in the bodies of those with switched cerebral asymmetry may be the best evidence that the brain masterminds body functions in ways that no scientist yet understands. Geschwind believes it is the endocrinology of the brain – its response to testosterone – that begins this cascade.

Brain/body relationships have been more closely studied by Herbert Benson who, more than any other Western scientist, has given the ancient wisdom of the East scientific validity. In his book, *The Relaxation Response*, Benson has outlined how Westerners might take advantage of the new understanding of brain/body relationships. His laboratory studies demonstrate that the body can learn new patterns of reaction; this inner wisdom can heal disease as effectively as a doctor's prescription.

Only recently have those in the West come to know of the benefits of meditation, but to those in the East the power of mind control is well accepted. With our knowledge of paracrinology, stories such as this one take on an exciting new significance:

The burial alive of the Yogi 'Haridas' in 1837 was authentically corroborated by Sir Claude Wade, Dr Jonos Honiberger and the British Consul at Lahore. Reports state that Haridas took only milk for several days before his burial. On the day of his burial he ate nothing, but performed the Yogic internal cleansing method of swallowing a long strip of cloth, retaining it for a while in the stomach to absorb bile, etc. Then he performed another internal cleansing exercise, nauli, standing up to his neck in warm water and washing out the colon. All the openings of his body were then stopped up with wax. As do many Yogis, he had cut the root of his tongue so that it could be rolled back to seal the entrance to the throat. Haridas was wrapped in linen and placed in a box which was locked by the Maharaja of Lahore and kept in a summer house with sealed door and windows. The house was guarded day and night by the Maharaja's body guard. After forty days the box was opened. The Yogi's servant washed his master with warm water, removed the wax stoppers and put warm yeast on his scalp. He forced the teeth open with a knife and unfolded the tongue. Tongue and eyelids then were rubbed with butter. After half-an-hour Haridas came to life, seemingly none the worse for his experience.

Unbelievable? If the nose had been stopped with wax, yes. If not, the Yogi's burial was little different from the hibernation of animals of many kinds.

A Western wiseman, Norman Cousins, employed the same technique to wake and rouse his tired and painful body:

I was coming unstuck. I had considerable difficulty moving my limbs and even turning over in bed. Nodules appeared on my body, gravel-like substances under the skin, indicating the systemic nature of the disease. At the low point of my illness, my jaws almost locked . . . I remembered having read, ten years or so earlier, Hans Selye's classic book, *The Stress of Life*. With great clarity, Selye showed that adrenal exhaustion could be caused by emotional tension, such as frustration or supressed rage. He detailed the negative effects of the negative emotions on body chemistry. The inevitable question arose in my mind: what about positive emotions? If negative emotions produce negative chemical changes in the body, wouldn't positive emotions produce positive chemical changes? Is it possible that love, hope, faith, laughter, confidence, and the will to live have therapeutic value? Do chemical changes occur only on the downside? Obviously, putting the positive emotions to work was nothing so simple as turning on a garden hose. But even a reasonable degree of control over my emotions might have a salutary physiologic effect . . . We were . . . able to get our hands on some old Marx Brothers films. We pulled down the blinds and turned on the machine. It worked. I made the joyous discovery that ten minutes of belly laughter had an anaesthetic effect and would give me at least two hours of painfree sleep. When the pain-killing effect of the laughter wore off, we would switch on the motion-picture projector again, and not infrequently, it would lead to another pain-free sleep interval.

And from Baghir Mostofi, the geologist from Iran who drilled the world's most productive oil well:

I was on my first job to locate and drill a deep-water well which I hoped would prove to be artesian. The region was swampy land south of Teheran, Iran, and full of mosquitoes. I soon found myself feverish. My temperature came like a clock, every second day, for weeks. With each fever came chills and malaise that sent me to my tent like a wounded hound. I knew I had contracted malaria but as the leader of the crew and on my first assignment no one else would know. By my interpretation of the subsurface geology we were above water but our well was as dry as dust. Several days went by. No water but many malarial fevers. We were on the last day of drilling as we were reaching the limit of our rig's capacity. I sensed I was going to have a dry hole on my hands and retired to my tent with a deep feeling of despair. An hour or so later one of the crew roused me with the news 'water'. I rushed from my tent and busied myself with controlling the artesian flow which is such a delight to watch. My joy was immense. Weeks, in fact months, went by before I realized that an external gush of water had produced an internal gush of joy by which I was healed. I received no other therapy, yet had not even one malarial fever after that joyful event.

Scientists have no idea what 'hormones of hibernation' were activated by the Yogi, what 'hormones of happiness' were released by Cousins's bouts of belly laughter, or what 'hormones of healing' gushed into Mostofi, but miracles of inner healing are everyday occurrences.

When scientists believed that the mind was driven by electricity, they asked priests and mystics to explain such miracles. But now, as scientists begin to acknowledge that hormonal harmonies regulate both the brain and the body, they look at these miracles with new interest. These anecdotes are not religious myths; they are 'true' and fit the scientific facts of the new paradigm. What are lacking are certain correlations between the offending illness and the healing hormone.

A decade ago I wrote an article in the *New England Journal of Medicine* entitled 'Neurosurgery May Die'. In it I lamented the lack of interest in brain research among my colleagues and criticized a system of education that resembled a factory that stamped out car fenders; students, like fenders, were all bent into the same shape. Many readers, especially neurosurgical educators, contended that my article overemphasized problems and neglected the description of opportunities. One wrote: 'Next time swing with the sharp side of the axe.'

Now I am filled with optimism about the future of my specialty, largely because of the development of endocrine neurology. This new medical science should bring together all those concerned with the brain in the same way that the NASA moonshot programme brought together many diverse groups. But because of the importance of the ventricles to the diagnosis and therapy of hormonally related brain illnesses, neurosurgeons may have the central role to play; they are the only people who are qualified to place catheters in human brains. Psychologists, psychiatrists and neurologists who want to know what is wrong with their patients will need neurosurgical help both to retrieve and replace the hormones in the hollow brain gland.

Young neurosurgeons, trained to believe that the operating microscope is the be all and end all of brain surgery, may find it difficult to accept that molecules, more than microscopes, will determine their future. Yet, more than any other medical or surgical specialty, neurosurgery now has the opportunity to join the revolution going on in molecular biology.

This brave new world will demand that those making the surgical decisions have a thorough knowledge of brain endocrinology. That knowledge now rests in the heads of those who live in basic science laboratories, and there will be no benefit to patients without educational strategies that carry this information into the heads of physicians, nurses, administrators and legal watchdogs. What is most important, patients must come to know and believe that a bold aggressive attack on the problems of the mind is not a fanciful fiction but a modern reality. Very special kinds of educational ploys may be required to educate people about the significance of brain hormones and the potential benefit that these substances could bring them and their relatives.

Before the mining and mending of brain hormones can begin, many fences must be torn down that separate physicians who care for patients with brain illnesses. Similar fences existed only a decade or two ago between those who cared for patients with heart disease, yet the unprecedented co-operation between all of those involved – cardiologists, radiologists, surgeons, and anaesthetists – yielded a benefit that has touched the lives of most of us.

There can be only one sharply focused goal for this new effort: improved patient care. For that to occur new consortiums must be developed for those who care for patients with hormone-related brain illnesses. One possible arrangement is shown in Fig. 15.1. This flow chart demonstrates how a patient with a particular brain hormone problem could he identified, referred, diagnosed, treated and evaluated. The chart emphasizes that no single group can begin this new effort alone; it requires co-operation from all involved. In the medical care of the brain, as in the scientific understanding of it, specialization can only yield so much benefit. At some point things have got to come together again.

The starting premise of the new knowledge that the brain is a gland is one of unity: the brain is one with the body. Its final observation is one of harmony: hormones come together to do the brain's bidding.

Unity must also be the starting premise of the clinicians who come together to develop new ways to treat those with brain diseases. But the physicians and scientists who focus on the brain must develop more harmonious relationships with radiologists, anaesthetists, pathologists, institutional administrators, third party insurance agents, and the legal profession before any of this can move forward.

There are two major legal problems surrounding the new opportunity to understand the significance of brain hormones to brain dysfunction: patient consent and malpractice.

Patients with severe brain problems are unable to sign legal documents, including consent forms for surgical procedures. Appropriately, courts protect the interests of these people

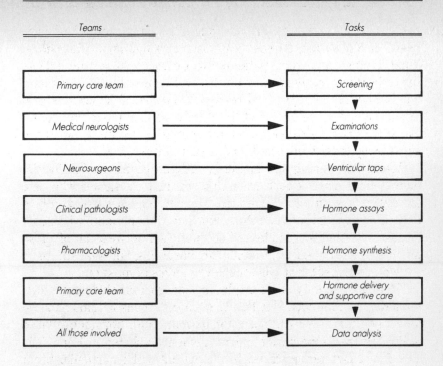

Fig. 15.1 A flow chart of care for patients with endrocrine abnormalities of the brain

because they are the easy prey of unscrupulous aggressors. Physicians, armed with the most noble interests in helping such patients, may be deterred from simple procedures such as drawing blood or performing spinal taps; the court says clearly and correctly, 'These patients shall not be guinea pigs.' In this setting, the suggestion of placing a diagnostic needle into the centre of the brain in such patients produces a shudder in the people who run psychiatric hospitals. The irony for these patients is that they may be cured of the brain malady that takes away their legal independence, but the law makes the first step impossible.

What is more important, perhaps, is the threat of malpractice. The legal umbrella that is intended to serve and protect the doctor-patient relationship now limits everyone concerned with the link between brain hormones and behavioural illnesses. Given the current malpractice climate, the knowledge that most of those who sit in jury boxes hold to the ancient notion that the brain is 'divine', and the sinister motivations that were attached to psychosurgeons less than a decade ago, few people are willing to take the risks inherent in these explorations.

The people who might back this new endeavour live in such fear of the legal consequence of a failed risk that they refuse to participate in what could be one of the most exciting and beneficial areas in medicine. With one eye on the patient and the other eye on the judge, they have tacitly cautioned all of those who might be involved, 'Accept the Dandy paradigm: measure pressure, not peptides; manipulate brain pressure, not brain peptides.'

Neurosurgeons will be involved most closely in the patient manipulations needed to link brain hormones to brain dysfunction. Consequently, the risks of these explorations, especially the malpractice risks, will fall very squarely upon our shoulders. These risks are not insurmountable, and I live with the belief that our society, once enlightened, will support the exploration of the mind and the risks entailed, as they have supported the exploration and the risks that astronauts have taken as they moved our society into space.

Consider how a new consortium of physicians, the one shown in Fig. 15.1, might handle the problems of your aunt, called 'Nellie'. You note that Nellie is not remembering things very well; she does well with the remote memories of her childhood, but her short-term memory is very bad. The first time you take Nellie to her physician, he examines her and says that she is ageing more rapidly than most. In the weeks that follow her memory becomes worse, so much worse that you seek medical attention again. On this visit the physician agrees that Nellie, at fifty-six, is in trouble and suggests she have psychological testing.

The psychologist's tests suggest that Nellie has an organic brain problem; she needs a neurologist, you are told.

After a more detailed examination, both a CAT scan and an NMR scan, the neurologist says that Nellie has 'presenile dementia'; there is nothing that can be done, you are told, and as you leave the office you are assured that she will not comprehend her suffering.

If this fate should befall Nellie this year, the neurologist would humanely suggest that you put both your anxieties and Nellie away.

If the disaster should befall Nellie in a year or two, I have little doubt that the neurologist will push for the measurement of ventricular peptides, and Nellie will have a ventricular tap.

Neurosurgeons perform ventricular taps with great frequency. In children with large ventricles this is easily done, but in adults with smaller ventricles the target is smaller and it is more difficult to tap the ventricle with confidence that the needle will pass directly into the ventricle. But the CAT scanner can guide the placement of the needle directly into the ventricle with little chance of error. Such a procedure is done under local anaesthesia, requires only a tiny incision and a drill hole into the skull to allow a delicate needle to be guided through the silent portion of the right brain into the right lateral ventricle. While this is not something to be done lightly, the risks are no greater than those for cardiac catheterization

Twenty years from now, the disease, 'presenile dementia' will be understood as well as diabetes is today. An insulin lack is presumed, though often not measured, in patients with diabetes. In decades to come, the confidence of the doctors looking after those like Nellie might grow to such an extent that they can predict Nellie's molecular problem. But for the next few years, until the molecular correlations are fully understood, the fluid removed from Nellie's brain will be sent to a laboratory for analysis.

Two kinds of tests will be performed on Nellie's brain fluid. The first will involve a screening test; at present the best such procedure is the two-dimensional gel study that separates molecules according to their electrical charges and their molecular weight. This test can count the number of different molecules in the fluid, but cannot determine the quantity of any of them.

A single drop of Nellie's ventricular fluid is all that is required for this test, yet it might yield a picture like that in Fig. 13.7. The pathologist who performs the two-dimensional gel study is very excited. His practised eye can quickly see that one spot is missing in Nellie's gel study. By comparing Nellie's brain fluid to that of other normal patients, the pathologist can tell precisely what substance Nellie lacks; his previous experience has taught him that the missing spot in the two-dimensional gel is 'x' hormone.

If the two-dimensional gel study showed a lack of 'x' hormone, the pathologist would predictably perform a second test that would measure quantitatively the amount of 'x' hormone in Nellie's ventricular fluid. This test, a 'radioimmune assay', can measure infinitesimal amounts of hormones in blood or other fluid with great specificity. The final report might read like this: "The concentration of 'x' hormone in the fluid is 31 nanograms per millilitre; in normal patients the concentration of 'x' hormone averages 243 nanograms per millilitre."

Of course, no one has performed two-dimensional gel studies on the ventricular fluid of patients with senile dementia. Therefore, no one knows for certain that Nellie would have an abnormal two-dimensional gel pattern. And it is unlikely that such studies will be performed in the current legal climate. But if the memory loss of presenile dementia is caused by a hormone deficiency and if pathologists in years to come can verify a lack of a memory hormone in this all-too-common disease, an opportunity for therapy would exist. If a 'memory peptide' could be found to be deficient in patients with senile dementia, these patients could be treated in the same way that patients with diabetes are treated with insulin.

The molecular structure of all of the known brain hormones is established, and genetic engineers already have begun bacterial production of most of them. Thus if a 'memory hormone' were found to be deficient in the brain of a patient such as Nellie, the synthetic hormone already might be on the pharmacist's shelf. If the memory loss of senile dementia were linked to a new brain hormone, genetic engineers would take this as a challenge and within a few months such a synthetic replacement could be available.

In this lies much of the excitement of the brain gland paradigm. Scientists have mastered the techniques of hormone analysis, measurement and manufacture. What is lacking is the correlation between a specific brain disease and a specific brain hormone. But scientists working alone cannot do this; these correlations can only come from a medical team of co-operating physicians.

If we assume that Nellie's problem with her memory can be linked with certainty to a particular hormone deficiency – a 'memory peptide' deficiency – and that this substance has been manufactured, how will it be given to Nellie?

As hers is a chronic illness, she will require 'memory peptide' for a long time, perhaps for the duration of her life, much as diabetics do. Some medicine can be given daily as a pill or capsule, but if 'memory peptide' is indeed a peptide it will be digested by the stomach. Conceivably, it could be given beneath the skin, as insulin is, but the presence of the blood-brain barrier makes it improbable that it would reach its target gland – the brain. Opening the blood-brain barrier at the same time that a particular drug is given would allow the drug to reach the brain, but only injections given into veins influence the blood vessels of the brain. Since Nellie's disease is chronic, daily intravenous injections are impractical if not impossible.

Everyone concerned would be led to the logical conclusion that Nellie's deficiency would be treated most effectively by giving 'memory peptide' where it is needed – in the brain itself. Again, since hers is a chronic illness, some delivery route must be organized that would allow daily, perhaps continuous, administration.

The same logic that led to the placement of the sampling catheter in the ventricle would lead to placing the delivery device in the ventricle, not the lumbar sac.

Animal experiments have confirmed the necessity of delivering hormones into the ventricle: the powerful hormone endorphin does not change behaviour if it is given intravenously; vasopressin will improve memory in animals only if it is given into the ventricles; insulin given through the bloodstream does not control appetite but is the best hormone for such control if given into the brain; and bombesin, an unusual substance found in frog skin, only stops stomach ulceration if given into the brain.

Everything we know about brain endocrinology points to the hollow spaces in the brain – the ventricles – as the best place for successful therapy.

A technique is available that may be used to deliver medication chronically into many organs of the body including the brain; it is shown in Fig. 15.2. Chronic infusion pumps are used every day in medical practice, generally in desperate situations such as cancer, but increasingly in the treatment of diabetes. The 'tanks' of these devices are placed beneath the skin, and the long catheter tip can be tunnelled long distances under the skin to the delivery site.

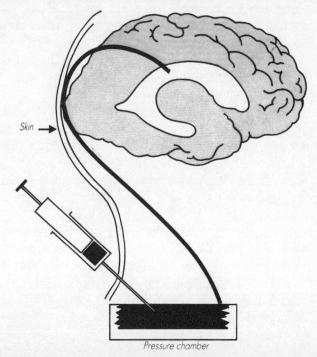

Skin →

Pressure chamber

Fig. 15.2 The 'infuse aid' allows long-term administration of drugs into different body spaces

Once or twice each month the 'tanks' in these devices are filled simply by sticking a delicate needle through the skin into the self-sealing rubber dome of the device.

Nellie's much needed 'memory peptide' could be placed into such a chronic pump and infused into the ventricles of her brain with very little technical difficulty. Even the rate of administration could be controlled.

Two more possibilities rest on the shelves of brain scientists: genetic manipulation and cell transplantation. Either of these could obviate the need for Nellie to have a chronic pump.

Genetic engineers predict that they soon will be able to manipulate the inside of human cells as easily as they now manipulate bacterial cells. Their best efforts so far have involved 'switching on' the production of specific hormones within cells, thus any deficiency disease that is identified in the brain would excite their interest. Much more research must be performed in animals before this is begun in patients, but tremendous strides have been taken by this group of scientists recently.

Genetic engineers are powerless in all of this without some co-operative effort from people working in allied fields. Certain correlations between a behavioural abnormality must precede the first thoughts about genetic manipulations, and again the importance of ventricular fluid for hormone analysis is apparent. It seems doubtful that the DNA-twisting 'wrenches' that they employ to bend genes back into shape would be effective across the blood-brain barrier; their manipulations may only be possible if they insert their wrenches through the ventricle.

Many of the best endocrine secrets were discovered by the simple expedient of moving one endocrine gland from one place to another, that is, by transplantation. When the brain was thought of as an electrically driven computer, there was no reason to believe that the transplantation of glandular tissue into the brain itself would modify behaviour, but now brain endocrinologists believe there is.

Already in animals, some gland-like cells have been transplanted from the adrenal gland into the brain, where they not only survive but continue their secretions. As brain diseases are linked more certainly to brain hormone deficiencies, such transplantations will be performed in humans. In nearly all other kinds of transplantations, donor organs or cells from other humans are employed; the body's immune system recognizes this tissue as foreign and attempts to get rid of it. Only suppression of the body's immunity to foreign substances will allow incompatible transplants to survive. Transplanting a tiny bit of a patient's own gland into his or her own brain sidesteps the problems of incompatibility and, because of this, gland transplants into the brain are viewed with optimism by transplant scientists (see Fig. 15.3).

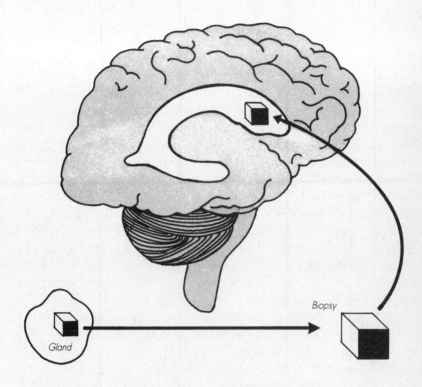

Fig. 15.3 Transplantation of gland tissue to the brain

Cellular biologists interested in transplantation have learned to harvest cells from endocrine organs in a way that allows a 'pure' population of a certain cell to be extracted from a certain organ. The six different kinds of cells in the pituitary, for example, can be separated into different populations and six 'soups' prepared, each containing a live population of one type of cell. The same thing can be done for many other endocrine organs.

By placing such cell-containing soup in bullet-shaped cell cages formed out of permeable plastics, a single population of cells can be introduced into the brain. The cells stay alive because the needed cell-food and life-giving oxygen penetrate the plastic envelope. By the same token, the hormones that are produced by the cells make their way through the surrounding permeable membrane into the brain. In this way, transplant scientists are able to create 'artificial glands' that can be inserted into specific regions of the brain with no fear of cell migration.

We have considered a disease, senile dementia, which might be associated with a hormone deficiency. But there are many other brain diseases that could be considered in the same way.

A fellow physician, while attending a patient who weighed more than 400 pounds, remarked, 'Four hundred pounds isn't too much, I once treated a man who weighed 700 pounds.' To which the lightweight replied, 'My goodness, how could he let himself *go* like that.' The anecdote suggests that obesity is a laughing matter, but malignant obesity is a disease with dire consequences and no cure. Increasingly, physicians and surgeons have recommended drastic surgical procedures, but none of these works very well and none is without severe side-effects. Malignant obesity stems from a disordered appetite, and the best evidence suggests that the control of appetite involves brain and gut hormones. Manipulating the appetite control centre in the brain is the most logical method of treatment and is certainly better than wiring the teeth together or re-routing the intestines. But until the hormonal control of the appetite centre is understood, such therapy cannot be considered.

As it is possible that the memory loss of senile dementia may stem from a deficiency of 'memory peptide', obesity may result from the deficiency of either bombesin, somatostatin, cholecystokinen, gastrin or insulin. As recorded in previous pages, animal studies make these relationships quite certain but, so far, human correlations are not possible. Again, as the hormones in the blood or in the lumbar fluid may not reflect what is going on inside the brain, it seems safe to predict that only ventricular measurements of these substances in humans can lead to certain correlations.

Many patients with schizophrenia, perhaps 20 per cent, have large ventricles that can be demonstrated by CAT or NMR scans. While such scans usually trigger the knee-jerk response for a ventricular shunt, to my knowledge shunts have not been performed for schizophrenic patients. Moreover, despite the evidence that ventricular hormones do not make their way out of the ventricle, the presence of large ventricles in many schizophrenic patients, and the ability of two-dimensional gels to provide a profile of peptides in the ventricle, not a single catheter has been placed into the ventricle of a schizophrenic patient to measure the peptides in the ventricle. This may be the most certain evidence that a legal roadblock exists that prevents the study of the relationship of brain hormones to brain diseases, for there is no logical reason why such studies should not have been done long ago.

Many endocrine diseases of the body entail the production of 'crooked molecules' – molecules that are made in the wrong way by the cell. It is fairly common for a cancer cell to begin the production of a 'crooked' hormone that evokes dramatic changes in other body functions.

Whether or not schizophrenia can be correlated with an excess of a hormone, a deficiency of a hormone, a crooked hormone, or no alteration in hormones at all is uncertain. But one thing is certain: as there is no animal model for this disease, the answer can only come from human studies.

Depression, more than any other human behavioural disorder, has clear-cut endocrine abnormalities. As many as one-half of the patients with unipolar depression have changes in the brain/ pituitary/adrenal axis that are so dramatic that they can be measured in the blood.

Cortisol, the hormone formed by the adrenal gland after it receives a command from the brain and pituitary, is typically elevated in the blood of these patients. While cortisol levels go up in the morning and down in the afternoon in normal people, in many who have a unipolar depression, such fluctuations are lost. If an attempt is made to shut down cortisol secretion by the administration of a synthetic hormone called 'decadron', it will be evident that the brain and pituitary are working overtime to stimulate cortisol secretion; decadron doesn't shut down production in a normal way.

Electroconvulsive therapy, or ECT, is the best therapy for unipolar depression that exists. It has been estimated that 10,000 patients still receive this therapy each day despite its bad press. Knowing that cortisol changes are correlated with mood in these patients allows doctors to monitor the effectiveness of electroconvulsive therapy; they have found that the smile will return to the face of the patient on the very same day that the cortisol dynamics return to normal. This new correlation promises to make the use of electroconvulsive therapy even more commonplace.

But why ECT is so effective remains a mystery. No one knows the cause of depression, despite its clear association with cortisol changes, but many people believe that if the effectiveness of ECT were understood, the cause of depression would be in hand.

Two things are certain: during electroconvulsive therapy the blood-brain barrier is opened and during the time that it remains opened there are heroically high levels of circulating pituitary hormones. Thus there is every reason to believe that this old-fashioned, poorly understood, and risky therapy is effective because it delivers hormones to the brain; it opens the brain's blood vessels with one hand while it whips the pituitary into action with the other. The brain under these conditions has little choice but to accept the hormones that come to it.

Opium was at one time used very effectively in the treatment of depression and some people contend that most of the therapies that have been effective in depression increase brain stores of brain opiates. Knowing that the pituitary contains great amounts of brain opiates has led to the speculation that ECT releases opiates – endorphins – which are manufactured in the pituitary and carried directly to the brain.

Some scientists contend that the changes in cortisol dynamics is evidence that the depressed brain is deficient in opiate hormones. They argue that an opiate-hungry brain demands that the pituitary secrete more opiate-like hormone; the cortisol excess seen in the bloodstream is only a reflection of a brain/pituitary relationship gone wrong.

Despite the effectiveness of electroconvulsive therapy, an improved rationale for its effectiveness, an endocrine test that allows physicians to monitor its effectiveness, and convincing evidence that ECT is given thousands of times daily, it may cause long-lasting problems with short-term memory. It is this risk which prevents it from being a panacea for those who are depressed, and it is this that has caused groups in our society to protest about its continued use. Yet despite the protests, the ability of cortisol studies to identify patients who will benefit from ECT guarantees that more patients will receive it.

The medical community in the best hospitals in the world would not allow a diagnostic ventricular tap for patients with senile dementia, obesity, schizophrenia or depression. 'It is too risky,' the doctors would say. But in these same hospitals far greater risks would be taken in patients whose epilepsy is not controlled by medications.

Patients with uncontrolled epilepsy have an evaluation that usually begins with electrical studies of the surface of the brain. Then electrodes are placed into the cheek to the space beneath the skull for recordings there. A hole is drilled in the skull, and electrical measurements made from within the depths of the brain. A large flap of the skull is then lifted up, electrodes placed on the surface of the brain, and the flap sewn back into place so that more electrical studies can be done.

The risks of these electrical tests are far greater than those associated with the ventricular taps needed for hormone studies, yet after this effort, and these risks, the team of physicians might say to the patient, 'We can't help.'

If the team of doctors say, 'We can help', they would detail which portions of the brain need to be excised. At operation the areas of the brain that are sending 'bad' electrical signals would be identified and removed. Rather large chunks of brain might be taken away in this process.

Somehow the same nurses, physicians, administrators and legal ombudsmen who prevented the study of the ventricular fluid of a patient with senile dementia, or obesity, or depression, or schizophrenia, because of the risks, will encourage diagnostic tests and therapy for patients with epilepsy that are far more destructive and immutable than the measurement and manipulation of hormones in the ventricle.

This may be one of the most glaring inconsistencies in medical practice; it is testimony to the institutional commitment to the old notion that electricity is the stuff of thought and verifies a fear of the new paradigm for the mind.

Must a brain disease be verified by electrical measurements before it can be rationally treated?

Is it 'legal' to accept the risk of a brain operation that measures the electrical currents in the brain and 'illegal' to accept the risk of a brain operation that measures the hormones in the brain?

May surgeons permanently modify the structural form of the brain but not transiently modify the structure of its molecules?

May electricity be pumped into the brain during ECT *knowing* that it causes memory loss, but hormones not be pumped into the brain because this therapy is too 'radical'?

The scientific discoveries of the past decade make it crucial that these questions be addressed; what must be done is fairly obvious. An informed public will demand fair-minded answers and actions from all those concerned with patient care, especially those who serve as advocates for 'patient's rights'.

It is more difficult to predict the impact of the new paradigm on other, non-medical aspects of our society. One thing seems certain: the hormonal genies that have lived unnoticed in the brain since humankind began have escaped; there is no way that they can be put back. No one can predict where they will go and what they will do.

The new stuff of thought, brain hormones, has a substance that is as sturdy as the planets. The exploration of the mind may begin with electrical studies, but electrically based technologies cannot shape the mind any more than they can shape outer space.

Space scientists have ended their efforts to know more about the surface of the moon and are now getting on with the task of shaping outer space in a way that will benefit people. Brain scientists can learn from this; they can also put aside their electrical gear and get on with the business of shaping the molecules of the mind. The high priests of brain exploration, like the high priests of space exploration, may continue to push for more electrical mapping studies of both the moon and the brain – their lives are made more secure by such studies – but it is difficult to see how the lot of the common man or woman is improved by either.

Is it unrealistic to believe that humankind's inner space – the mind – can be reshaped with the same gusto and co-operation which led to the reshaping of earth's outer space? I think not.

Look back for a moment to the 1945 'Wireless World' predictions of Arthur C. Clarke. He foretold the moonshot, communications satellites, the exploration of far distant planets and the space shuttle. Many stored his predictions on the same shelves as the Buck Rogers futuristic comics, but his notions were the prescient predictions for space explorations.

Aristrachus, Copernicus, Galileo and Kepler were merely spectators of man's outer space. They used their visual sense and optical telescopes to make observations that were fundamentally correct; the electronic signals from our satellites have shown these ancient geniuses to be correct in almost every way.

Einstein, Goddard, Arthur C. Clarke and John Glenn were not mere spectators; they actually reshaped people's outer space. They forswore the descriptive telescope, either optical or radio-based, and grappled with new issues – gravitational forces, rocket propellants, the magic of the satellite and the Gs that the human body could withstand to place people in space and eventually on the moon. The passive spectator-like study of space gave little benefit to mankind; the active athletic-like reshaping of space – John Glenn's willingness to ride on a rocket, for example – provided humankind immense benefit.

Brain scientists now stand on a threshold very similar to that of space scientists. They recognize the similarities between our outer and our inner spaces; the spinning molecules within the human mind are very much like the spinning planets that make up our universe. Electrically based studies must begin each kind of exploratory endeavour but, at the end, only the physical reshaping of each will benefit mankind.

Our outer macrocosm already has been partly reshaped by rocketing small chunks of earth – metal communications satellites – into orbit. The inner microcosm – the human mind – can also be reshaped by nudging the molecules of the mind, brain hormones, into new orbits.

But not quickly. The complexities of the hormonal harmonies which modulate the mechanisms of the mind secure the prediction that endocrine studies of mind/body correlations will go on for many centuries. The lengthy commitment that research and health care institutions have made to brain electricity – a commitment that has not given either those who are well or those who are sick any great advantages – should pall as those concerned come to see the opportunities that brain hormones bring to the understanding of normal and abnormal human behaviour.

Arthur C. Clarke said in 1945, 'Humans *will* launch satellites, they *will* go to the moon, and they *will* live in space.' His only question was, '*When?*'

In 1984, parallel predictions are in order: physicians and scientists *will* measure brain hormones – in ventricular fluid and elsewhere – *will* link these to specific diseases, and *will* devise space-age techniques to restock the mind's hormonal pantries. The only question is, '*When?*'

Those who care for patients with brain illness – psychologists, psychiatrists, neurologists, neurosurgeons, and family physicians – suddenly find themselves at the cutting edge of molecular biology. Suddenly, these doctors are positioned between scientists with potential 'cures' and patients with 'incurable' brain diseases. Their schools, postgraduate training programmes, current leaders and journals have not prepared them for this new role.

In medicine this is unprecedented, but it might be the predictable consequence of a rapidly developing new science making an impact on a broadly educated public and a narrowly educated group of professionals.

In 1945 Arthur C. Clarke was forced to write his 'Wireless World' predictions in a manner and in a place that were accessible to the public, and decades passed before the space race became a reality. During that interval, most, if not all, aviators learned about space travel from newspaper comic strips. Before the moonshot, whole new strategies of education were developed to get the young and old space adventurers upgraded and ready for space travel.

The new knowledge about brain hormones is in every way like the 1945 knowledge about space travel. For mankind to benefit from this new brain information whole new strategies of education must be developed to upgrade those who provide health care. Without that effort, the new knowledge about the brain will rest on laboratory benches and library shelves.

For millions who are ill, the realization that the brain is a hormonally modulated gland is revolutionary therapeutic good news. But as long as our most respected ombudsmen maintain Plato's belief in a 'divine' brain, and as long as that view creates the legal climate that allows physicians to manipulate the pressure and electricity in the brain but not manipulate its peptide hormones, little of the potential benefit of the brain gland revolution will be realized.

Those who keep the 'truth' at the centre of the island of knowledge must now contemplate the wealth of new information about the mind coming from the 'truthfinders' at the shoreline of wonder. The new pathfinders describe a pattern for the fabric of the mind that is woven of many kinds of thread. They say that a single strand may be pulled out, analysed and synthesized, and that such new braids may even be rewoven into the fabric of the mind if mending is required. Truthkeepers might easily accept all of these new scientific discoveries about brain hormones – they involve reductions, indeed abbreviations, and left brains brought together find such things both comprehensible and teachable.

But how will those who keep the 'truth' deal with the evidence that the thoughts emerging from the mind spring from hormonal harmonies – from molecules of many kinds coming together in many places? Will they recognize the cosmic entity that orchestrates the anatomical trysts of the hormones that steer the mind? Predictably, no. Reductionists – especially those banded in a group – will not see it.

Yet the pattern-discerning right brain of any individual who takes the time to understand the new make-up of thought will be forced to the conclusion that the fabric of the mind is woven by some wise creator. Those who discern the pattern of the tapestry will stand in awe, knowing that its static form cannot produce thought: molecules, some from the brain and others from the body, must caress each other – as the violinist's bow kisses the violin strings – to create the music of the mind.

What force moves these molecules?

Out of that question can grow a new beginning.

Akil, D., Mayer, D. J. and Liebeskind, J. D., 'Antagonism of Stimulation-produced Analgesia by Naloxone, a Narcotic Antagonist', *Science*, 191, 961–2, 1976. [This article was published one year after the discovery of opiate-like hormones in the brain and suggested that the 'gate-control' of pain was mediated by hormones.]

Altschule, M., *Origins of Concepts in Human Behavior*, Wiley, New York, 1977. [This little book set me on the historical trail of the stuff of thought.]

Aristotle, *De Partibus Animalium*, in *The Works of Aristotle* [translated by W. Ogle] Clarendon Press, London, 1912.

Berger, H.,'Das Electrenkephalogramm des Menschen', *Acta Nova Leopolda*, 6, 173, 1938. [The classic description of the EEG.]

Bergland, R., 'New Information Concerning the Irish Giant', *Journal of Neurosurgery*, 23, 265–9, 1965. [This tells how the father of general surgery, John Hunter, and the father of neurosurgery, Harvey Cushing, collaborated in the evaluation of the giant, Charles O'Brien.]

Bergland, R., 'Neurosurgery May Die', *New England Journal of Medicine*, 288, 1043–6, 1973. [A controversial article espousing my belief that neurosurgeons should be more involved in research.]

Bergland, R., Ray, B. S. and Torack, R., 'Anatomical Variations in the Human Pituitary Gland . . . (225 autopsies), *Journal of Neurosurgery*, 28, 93–9, 1968.[It was while doing this work that I came to believe that pituitary hormones might flow 'north' to the brain.]

Bergland, R. and Torack, R., 'Follicular Cells in the Human Pituitary'; *American Journal of Pathology*, 57, 273–98, 1969. [The first description of these cells in humans.]

Bergland, .R. and Torack, R., 'An Electronmicroscopic Study of the Human Infundibulum', *Zeitschrift fur Zellforschung*, 99, 1–12, 1969. [For this work I saved bits of the pituitary stalk that I had removed during hypophysectomy. It demonstrates neurosecretory granules produced by the brain – little 'balls' within axons.]

Bergland, R., 'Neurosecretory Bodies within the Median Eminence in association with Pituitary Tumors', *Lancet*, 2, 1270–2, 1979. [The first description of this association.]

Bergland R., and Page, R. B., 'Can the Pituitary Secrete Directly to the Brain? (Affirmative Anatomical Evidence)', *Endocrinology*, 102, 1325–38, 1979. [Bob Page and I studied pituitary vascular casts in eleven species; this article pertains to the rhesus monkey and challenges many of the 'holy' concepts in neuroendocrinology.]

Bergland, R. and Page, R. B., 'Pituitary-Brain Vascular Relations: a New Paradigm', *Science*, 204, 18–24, 1979. [This article questions the concept that the pituitary gland always sends its secretions 'south' to the body and shows many mechanisms which can carry hormones 'north' to the brain.]

Bergland, R. M., *et al*, 'ACTH may be Transported directly to the Brain', *Science*, 210, 541–3, 1980. [At least during ECT in sheep, this happens.]

Bernard, C., 'Lecons sur la Physiologie et la pathologie du systeme nerveux', *Bailliere*, Paris, 1858. [The father of physiology, writing the first textbook of physiology. In it he espouses the importance of chemical studies for the body but accepts Schwann's view that the brain is driven by electricity.]

Bernard, C., *Cahier Rouge* [English translation], Shenkman, Cambridge, Massachusetts, 1967. [In this little bedside notebook we learn that Bernard thought the brain was a gland, yet in his daytime lectures he taught the 'network theory'.]

Beumont, P. J. V. and Burrows, G. D., *Handbook of Psychiatry and Endocrinology*, Elsevier, Amsterdam, 1982. [This is a good correlation between psychiatric diseases and hormone abnormalities.]

Black, P. M., 'Neuropeptides in Cerebrospinal Fluid', Neurosurgery, 11, 550–5, 1982. [Review.]

Blakemore, C., *Mechanics of the Mind*, Cambridge University Press, Cambridge 1977. [Certainly the best illustrated popular book about the brain. It contains a good description of Plato's *mismeme* about males and females.]

Bloom, F. E., 'Neuropeptides', *Scientific American*, 245, 148–168, 1981. [A publication which explains all the rudiments of brain endocrinology.]

Bloom, F. E., 'The Functional Significance of Neurotransmitter Diversity', *American Journal of Physiology, 241, C184 194, 1984.*

Bloom, F., *et al*, 'Endorphins: Profound Behavioural Effects, Science', 194, 630–4, 1976. [Describes 'catatonia' in rats, but only after the ventricular administration of endorphin.]

Bogan, J. E., 'The Other Side of the Brain', *Bulletin of the Los Angeles Neurological Society*, 34, 135–62, 1969.[Joe Bogan, a neurosurgeon, describes the 'corpus callosum divisions' that he did in patients with epilepsy. These patients were crucial to Roger Sperry's work on the right and left brain.]

Bradshaw, R., 'Nerve Growth Factor', *Annual Review of Biochemistry*, 47, 191–216, 1978. [Bradshaw describes how nerve-growth factor can penetrate cell membranes and be carried by retrograde axonal flow to the nucleus of the nerve cell.]

Brightman, M. W. and Reese, T. S., 'Junctions between Apposed Cells in the Brain', *Journal of Cell Biology*, 40, 648–77, 1969. [These authors show that horseradish peroxidase placed into the ventricle leaks into the brain. If horseradish peroxidase does this, water most certainly does. This challenges the central premise of the Dandy paradigm for brain water which contends that water is made in the choroid plexus and flows out of the ventricle.]

Brightman, M. W. and Rosenstein, J. M., 'Cerebrospinal Fluid Compartment as Site for Neural Transplantation', *Frontiers in Hormone Research*, 9, 36–50, 1982. [Nerve ganglia, moved into the ventricle, lack a blood-brain barrier, these authors note. Such manoeuvres could provide a 'back door' by which hormones could be delivered to the brain.]

Bronowsky, J., *The Ascent of Man*, British Broadcasting Corporation, London, 1973. [This famous book details the technological stepping-stones of civilization's ascent. Yet the history of mankind has not been a continual ascent. In AD 200 it took a nosedive. Why? While Bronowsky bypasses the question of the 'descent of man', I blame Galen (AD 130–200).]

Brushart, T. M. and Mesulam, M., 'Connections between Muscle and Anterior Horn Cells', *Science*, 208, 603–5, 1980. [This article (and the *Science* cover) show that horseradish peroxidase, injected into leg muscles, is carried by nerve fibres into the spinal cord.]

Calvin, W. H. and Ojemann, G. A., *Inside the Brain*, New American Library, New York, 1980. [This little-known book describes in lay terms what epilepsy surgery is all about.]

Carr, D., Bergland, R. M. *et al.*, 'Endotoxin-stimulated Opioid Peptide Secretion . . . , *Science*, 217, 845–8, 1982. [This study of febrile sheep shows heroic elevations of endorphin during fever. This may explain the 'delirium' which accompanies illnesses which cause elevated body temperature.]

Coghlan, J., *et al*, 'Hybridization Histochemistry: Use of Recombinant DNA for Tissue Localization of Specific Messenger RNA Populations', *Clinical and Experimental Hypertension; Theory and Practice*, 6, 63–78, 1984. [The first description of this technique.]

Copernicus, Nicolai, *De Revolutionibus Orbium Coelestium*, Nuremberg, 1543. [One of the most important books in the history of thought. It gives the first 'true' cosmological description of our outside world – of Aristotle's macrocosm. Remarkably, this was published in the same year as Vesalius's *Fabric of Man*, which gives the first 'true' anatomical description of our inner world – of Aristotle's microcosm.]

Cousins, N., *The Anatomy of an Illness*, Norton, New York, 1978. [A description of the healing power of joy.]

Cox, B., 'Endogenous Opioid Peptides; a Guide to Structure and Terminology', *Life Sciences*, 31, 1645–58, 1982. [This documents, in orderly fashion, the endorphin situation as it was in 1982.]

Cushing, Harvey, The Bio-bibliography of Andreas Vesalius, Archon, Hamden, Connecticutt, 1962. [Compiled twenty-three years after Cushing's death by John Fulton and friends.]

Cushing, H., 'Removal of a Subcortical Tumour without Anaesthesia', *Journal American Medical Association*, 1, 847, 1908. [The first

description of a 'cortical map' in a human, written two decades before
Penfield.]

Cushing, H., *The Pituitary Body and Its Disorders*, Lippincott, Philadelphia, 1912. [Maybe the most important scientific book written by a
modern surgeon. It is here that Cushing gives his reasons for believing
the pituitary is the 'conductor of the endocrine orchestra'.]

Cushing, H., *Studies in Intracranial Physiology*, Oxford University
Press, 1926.

Cushing, H., 'The Third Circulation and its Channels', *Lancet*, 209, 851,
1925. [The questions Cushing sets down here challenge the Dandy
paradigm and have never been answered.]

Cushing, H., 'The Reaction of Posterior Pituitary Extract when Injected
into the Ventricles', *Proceedings of the National Academy of Science*,
17, 163–80, 239–64, 1931. [Intuitively, Cushing thought that the
pituitary must secrete to the brain and performed these bold experiments in humans.]

Dale, H., 'Chemical Transmission of the Effects of Nerve Impulses',
British Medical Journal (May issue), 1934. [Note the absence of Feldberg's name, yet it was Feldberg's assay that allowed the work.]

Dandy, W. E. and Blackfan, K. D., 'An Experimental and Clinical Study of
Internal Hydrocephalus, *Journal of the American Medical Association*, 61, 2216, 1913. [The description of the legendary 'aqueductal
obstruction' experiments.]

Dandy, W. E., 'Internal Hydrocephalus. An Experimental, Clinical and
Pathological Study', *American Journal of Diseases of Children*, 8,
406–82, 1914. [Here Walter Dandy records the results of choroid
plexus removal.]

Dandy, W. E., *The Brain* [2nd edn], Prior, Hagerstown, Maryland, 1966.
[In this classic, Dandy describes the operations he advocated for the
treatment of hydrocephalus.]

Dawkins, R., *The Selfish Gene*, Oxford University Press, Oxford, 1976.
[The last chapter of this book describes memes, or ideas that pass from
brain to brain like an infectious virus. My new word, 'mismemes', or
'wrong' ideas that pass from brain to brain, came from Dawkins's
neologism.]

de Robertis, E. D. P., 'Submicroscopic Morphology of the Synapse',
Experimental Cell Research, supplement 5, 347–69, 1958. [The first
clear-cut demonstration of the synaptic cleft and synaptic vesicles.]

de Wied, D. and van Keep, P. A., *Hormones and the Brain*; Mather
Brothers; Preston, England, 1980. [de Wied has done more to demon-
strate the importance of peptides to memory than any other scientist.
This reviews that experience.]

Della-Ferra, M. A., *et al*, 'Peptides with CCK-like Activity Administered
Intracranially Elicit Satiety in Sheep', *Physiology of Behaviour*, 26,
979–83, 1981. [Cholecystokinen – CCK – limits appetite in sheep only
if given into the ventricle.]

Descartes, R., *De Homine Figuris et Latinate Donatus a Florentio
Schuyl*, Frances Moyard and Peter Leff, Leyden, 1662. [This book
demonstrates that Descartes was not an accurate anatomist.]

Doby, T., *Discoverers of Blood Circulation*, Abelard-Schuman; London, 1963. [Wonderfully illustrated; the most readable account of the meme that passed from Vesalius to Fabricius to Harvey.]

du Vigneaud, V., 'Trail of Sulfur Research from Insulin to Oxytocin', *Science*, 123, 967, 1956. [For the work described here du Vigneaud won the Nobel Prize.]

Eccles, J. C., The Understanding of the Brain, McGraw-Hill; New York, 1973. [Eccles articulates in this book the long-accepted view that electricity is the stuff of thought. No modern neurophysiologist has done as much as Eccles. His belief that the 'mind' is more than the sum of the parts of the brain should have fuelled the furnaces of the 'holists' more than it has.]

Eccles, J. C., 'The Effects of Nerve Cross-union on Muscle Contraction', in *Exploratory Concepts in Muscular Dystrophy*, Excerpta Medica, Amsterdam, 1966. [This is the first description of genes 'switching on' in response to commands from the brain.]

Edwards, B., *Drawing on the Right Side of the Brain*, Tarcher; New York, 1979. [Even brain scientists can learn something from this light, well-written work of an art teacher.]

Eng, R., Shapiro, R. and Miselis, R., 'Vagal Afferents to the Area Postrema', *Neuroscience Abstracts*, 8, 273, 1982. [A description of the flow of horseradish peroxidase from the stomach through the vagus nerve to the brain stem – an important but little known non-electrical link between the nervous system and the gut. Knowing that the gut contains brain hormones raises the question, 'Can gut hormones move to the brain via this route?']

Engeland, W. C. and Dallman, M. F., 'Compensatory Adrenal Growth is Neurally Modulated', *Neuroendocrinology*, 19, 352–62, 1975. [This paper confirms what Halasz and Szentagothai reported in 1969: there are non-electrical 'commands' coming from the brain to the endocrine system along specific pathways.]

Erlanger, J. and Gasser, H., 'The Compound Nature of the Action Current of Nerve', *American Journal of Physiology*, 70, 624–66, 1924. [For this paper these authors won the Nobel Prize.]

Fabricius ab Aquapendente, *De Venarum Ostiollis*, L. Pasquati, Padua, 1603. [The drawings in this book – mirror-images of those employed in 1628 by Harvey – confirm that it was important to Harvey's discovery of the circulation.]

Feldberg, W. S., *Fifty Years On: Looking Back On Neurohumoral Physiology*, Liverpool University Press, 1982. [Few have done more pioneering work in the nervous system than Feldberg. This describes much of it. Neurosurgeons who tinker in the posterior fossa should note this article carefully.]

Feyrter, F., *Ueher die peripheren Endokrinen (Paracrinen) Druesen des Menschen*, Maudrick, Wien-Duesseldorf, 1953. [Feyrter first proposed 'paracrine' relations in 1938, yet the term 'paracrinology' was popularized most by Guillemin in 1978.]

Franklin, Benjamin, '*Letter to Peter Collinson, Philadelphia, October 19,*

1752'; Reprinted in *Ben Franklin: New World Physicist*, Pergamon Press, 1973. [Two pages that changed the world.]

Frederickson, R. C. and Geary, L. E., 'Endogenous Opioid Peptides: A Review, *Progress in Neurobiology*, 19, 19–69, 1982. [This review notes that 7,500 papers pertaining to endogenous opiates were published between 1976 and 1981. It contains the best endorphin/enkephalin bibliography I have seen.]

Fulton, J. F., *The Biography of Harvey Cushing*, Thomas Springfield, 1946. [Anyone who reads this will stand in awe of Cushing who is without peer in the history of American medicine, science, education, communications and patriotism. Cushing built a surgical specialty – neurosurgery – a fundamental science – neuroendocrinology – a hospital – Peter Bent Brigham at Harvard – and a library at Yale. Yet he had time to go to war – twice – and write many books, one of which won the Pulitzer Prize and several which remain classics.]

Fulton, J. F., *Selected Readings in the History of Physiology*, Thomas, Springfield, 1966. [This is a model for those who write about the history of science.]

Fulton, J. F., *Micheal Servetus, Humanist and Martyr*, Herbert Reichner, New York, 1953. [It was John Calvin's church, not the Catholic church, that demanded the death of Servetus.]

Galen, Claudius, *Opera Omnia [Twenty-two volumes of translation]*, Nackdrunk der Ausgabe, Leipzig, 1821.[Don't read these volumes, just try to lift them. They are overwhelming by weight alone, and they held mankind in intellectual chains for 1,400 years.]

Galvani, Luigi, *De Viribus Electricitatis in Motu Musculari...*, Apud Societem Typographicam, Mutine, 1791. [The 'twitching frog legs' classic; interesting lithographs.]

Garfield, E. [ed.], *Current Contents* Philadelphia; published weekly. [Those who seek to correlate hormones with behaviour – either normal or abnormal – can find no better guiding periodical than this. Its back pages have been computer-indexed to make it easy. Scientists *must* have this to stay abreast of the many rapid changes in the endocrinology of the brain.]

Gazzinaga, M. S., 'The Split Brain of Man', *Scientific American*, 217, 24–9, 1967. [In this the kinds of tests that Roger Sperry employed in his 'left brain – right brain' work are described.]

Geren, B. B., 'The Formation from Schwann Cell Surfaces of Myelin', *Experimental Cell Research*, 7, 558–64, 1954. [In the early days of electronmicroscopy, Geren published this description of myelin formation. Only then did scientists realize that Schwann cells were wrapped around nerves in 'jelly-roll' fashion.]

Gerendai, I., *et al*, 'The Neural Pathway from the Adrenal Gland to the Hypothalamus', *Cell and Tissue Research*, 153, 559, 1974. [The continuation of the Halasz and Szentagothai experiments done first in 1959.]

Gerendai, I. and Scapagnini, U., 'Neural Mechanism and Ovarian Hypertrophy', *Proceedings of the International Symposium on Neuroendocrine Regulatory Mechanisms*, Belgrade, 101–5, 1979. [This describes how non-electrical, non-pituitary commands from the brain to control genetic mechanisms in the ovary.]

Geschwind, N., 'Specialization of the Human Brain', *Scientific American*, 241, 180–99, 1979.

Geschwind, N. and Behan, F., 'Left Handedness, Association with Immune Diseases, Migraine, and Developmental Learning Disorder', *Proceedings of the National Academy of Sciences*, 79, 5097–100, 1982. [Geschwind postulates here that testosterone imbalance in the brain causes all these things.]

Goldstein, A., Lowney, L. I. and Pal, B. K., 'Interaction of Morphine in Mouse Brain', *Proceedings of the National Academy of Science*, 68, 1742–9, 1971. [This contains the description of the 'opiate receptor' that led to the discovery of the endorphins.]

Golgi, C., 'Recherches sur l'histologie des centres nerveux', *Archives of Italian Biology*, 3, 285–317, 1883. [This contains Golgi's mismeme espousing the 'network theory' of the brain.]

Guillemin, R., 'Peptides in the brain: The New Endocrinology of the Neuron', *Science*, 202, 390–402, 1978. [Sir Isaac Newton, in a tribute to Kepler, said, 'If I have seen further, it is because I have stood on the shoulders of giants.' For the rest of time, all of those who think about thinking will stand on this article of Guillemin's, much as Newton stood on the writings of Kepler.]

Guillemin, R., Burgus, R. and W. Vale, 'The Hypothalamic Hypophysiotropic Thyrotropin Realeasing Factor', *Vitamins and Hormones*, 29, 1, 1971. [This is what Guillemin wrote about this work: '... we processed close to five million hypothalamic fragments from the brains of sheep. Since one sheep brain has a wet weight of about 100 grams, this meant handling 500 tons of brain tissue ... Finally in 1968 one milligram of a preparation of TRF was obtained.']

Halsted, W., 'Auto and Isotransplantation of Parathyroid Glands', *Journal of Experimental Medicine*, 11, 175, 1909. [Here Halsted notes that transplanted glands survive if the host glands are removed before transplantation. This observation was, in retrospect, the first demonstration of the 'feedback control' that underlies all endocrine relationships.]

Halasz, B. and Szentagothai, J., 'Histologischer Beweis einer Nervosen Signalubermittlung von der Nebennierenrinde zum Hypothalamus', *Zeitschrift fur Zellforschung*, 50, 297–306, 1959. [This article will someday be recognised as the keystone to the development of paracrinology, for it documents for the first time the non-electrical, non-pituitary neural connections between the brain and the endocrine system.]

Harvey, W., *Exercito Anatomica de Motu Cordis et Sanguinus in Animalibus*, William Fitzer, Frankfurt, 1628. [This book became the turning point for science, medicine, philosophy and religion. Yet it addressed a simple anatomical question, 'Why is the heart hollow?' Someday somebody will write a similar book which answers the simple question 'Why is the brain hollow?' Will that book have the same impact? I think so.]

Harris, G., *Neural Control of the Pituitary*, Arnold, London 1955. [This is Harris's finest written work and a classic.]

Harris, G., 'Humours and Hormones', *Proceedings of the Society for Endocrinology*, Dale lecure, ii–xxiii, 1971. [In this article Harris tells his story.]

Hewitt, J., *Yoga*, English Universities Press, 1960. [The quote about the hibernating yogi on page 160 came from this book.]

Hinsey, J., 'A Search for the Neurological Mechanisms of Ovulation', *Proceedings of the Society for Experimental Biology and Medicine*, 30, 136, 1932. [This article established that the brain controlled ovulation by chemical commands, and not by electrical signals. It is the foundation of neuroendocrinology, according to Meites and Medvei.]

Hodgkin, A. L. and Huxley, A. F., 'Currents Carried by Sodium and Potassium Ions ...', *Journal of Physiology*, 116: 449–72, 1952. [For this discovery the authors shared the Nobel Prize.]

Hofstadter, D. R., *Godel, Escher, Bach: An Eternal Golden Braid*, Harvester Press, London, 1979. [Godel used numbers, Escher used pictures and Bach used music. But Hofstadter uses words. All do the same thing: they examine the mysterious mechanisms of the mind.]

Hosubuchi, J., Rossier, J., Bloom, F. and Guillemin, R., 'Beta-endorphin in Ventricular Fluid', *Science*, 203, 279–81, 1979. [Hosubuchi, a neurosurgeon, implanted electrodes into the mid brains of patients with intractable pain much as Reynolds (see below) did in animals. When a current was passed through the electrodes, endorphin levels rose in ventricular fluid. This is a very important observation in the understanding of the fabric of the mind.]

Hughes, J., 'Isolation of an Endogenous Compound from the Brain with the Pharmacological Properties similar to Morphine, *Brain Research*, 88, 295–308, 1975. [Although this article was published without his name, Kosterlitz is regarded as the co-discoverer of brain opiates.]

Huxley, T. H., *Collected Essays*, Macmillan, London, 1906. [Has anyone written better? Or more? From Huxley came my quote about an island of knowledge.]

Huxley, T. H., 'On Certain Errors Respecting the Heart Attributed to Aristotle', *Nature*, 21, 1–5, 1880. [This article explains how Aristotle's 'hollow arteries' and his 'three-chambered heart, were the result of his insistence that animals be killed by strangulation.]

Katz, B., 'The Transmission of Impulses from Nerve to Muscle', *Proceedings of the Royal Society of London*, 155: 455–77, 1962. [For this Katz won the Nobel Prize.]

Kelsey, M. I., Hymer, W. C. and Page, R. B., 'Pituitary Cell Transplants to the Cerebral Ventricles Suppress the Pituitary', *Neuroendocrinology*, 33, 312–16, 1981.

Knight, B., *Discovering the Human Body*, Heinemann, London, 1980. [The best illustrated history of anatomical discovery that exists. Knight explains in detail the importance of Vesalius.]

Kobler, J., *The Reluctant Surgeon*, Doubleday, New York, 1960. [A very readable account of the life of John Hunter.]

Koestler, A., *The Sleepwalkers*, Hutchinson, London, 1959. [*Sleepwalkers*, more than any other book, shows how a wrong view of the macrocosm influenced the course of civilization. it stimulated me to wonder if a wrong view of the microcosm – of the stuff of thought – has done the same.]

Kreiger, D. T. and Liotta, A. S., 'Pituitary Hormones in Brain: Where, How and Why', *Science*, 205, 366–72, 1979. [Kreiger was the first to describe ACTH in the brain. She writes here that she is not convinced I am correct in stating that pituitary hormones may be carried to the brain.]

Kreiger, D. T., *et al.*, 'Brain Grafts Reverse Hypogonadism', *Nature*, 298, 468–71, 1982. [If I read the tea leaves correctly, this will be a historically important article.]

Kruseman, N., *et al.*, 'CRF in the Human Gastrointestinal Tract, *Lancet*, 2, 1245, 1982. [CRF was found first in the brain, but now it is found in many places. Kruseman's discovery of it in the gut came in the same year that Tanaka, and others, found 31-K in the gut. All kinds of evidence show that CRF and 31-K are important to thinking, especially to memory. Can the gut think?]

Kuhn, T. S., *The Structure of Scientific Revolutions*, University of Chicago press, 1962. [This book has mind-jarring insights into the thought processes that underlie new discoveries. It stresses the importance of paradigms and was the catalyst in my decision to write about the need for a paradigm switch.]

Lashley, K. S., 'Persistent Problems in the Evolution of the Mind', *Quarterly Review of Biology*, 24, 28–42, 1949; and 'In Search of the Engram', *Symposia of the Society of Experimental Biology*, 4, 454–82, 1950. [Lashley gained fame for performing rat experiments for twenty years searching for the site of memory. He couldn't find it. His acknowledgement of failure was important for those who would later claim that memory was a 'holographic' process.]

Li, C. H., *et al*, 'Isolation of Lipotropin from Sheep Pituitary Glands', *Nature*, 208, 1093–4, 1965. [Here, ten years before the discovery of endorphin and enkephalin, Li described the giant peptide lipotropin.]

Levi-Montalcini, R. and Angeletti, P. U., 'Nerve Growth Factor: Evaluation and Perspectives', In Zaimis E. (ed.) *Nerve Growth Factor*, Athlone, London, 1972. [Who would have thought that material from the salivary gland could be important to the nervous system? Levi-Montalcini made that discovery.]

Lewin, R., 'The Brain's Own Opiate', *New Scientist*, January, 1976. [Lewin, one of the world's best science writers, tells in this article about the serendipitous recognition that the molecular sequence of the brain hormone, enkephalin was present in Li's pituitary lipotropin.]

Lucion, A. B., *et al*, 'Intracerebroventricular Administration of Nanogram Amounts of Endorphin or Enkephalin Cause Retrograde Amnesia', *Behavioural Brain Research*, 4, 111–15, 1982. [First de Wied and his mates say that one end of the 31–K molecules *enhances* memory. Now comes this publication, saying that the other end of 31–K *limits* memory. Most important for clinicians who hope to modify the endocrine environment of the brain: both effects depend upon intraventricular, not intravascular, administration.]

Lund, R. D. and Hauska, S. D., 'Transplanted Neural Tissue to Rat Brain',

Science, 193, 582–4, 1976. [This is the first of many 'brain transplant' articles from this pace-setting Swedish group.]

MacCullum, W. G., *William Stewart Halsted,* Johns Hopkins Press, Baltimore, 1930. [There is a hidden side of Halsted that has not yet been written about, certainly not here.]

Mains, R. E., Eipper, B. A. and Ling, N., 'Common Precursor to Corticotropins and Endorphins', *Proceedings of the National Academy of Sciences*, 74, 3014–18, 1977. [This article describes 31–K – the giant prohormone in the pituitary gland.]

Mason, S. F., *A History of the Sciences*, Macmillan, New York, 1962. [Certainly the best single source book I found in my history of science research.]

McComb, J. G., 'Recent Research into the Nature of Cerebrospinal Fluid Formation and Absorption', *Journal of Neurosurgery*, 59, 369–83, 1983. [This is an excellent review article. It documents that very few scientists in 1983 question Dandy's paradigm for brain water which was advanced in 1911.]

Medawar, P. B., *Advice to a Young Scientist*, Harper and Row, London, 1979. [Also good advice for old scientists.]

Medawar, P. B., *Pluto's Republic*, Oxford University Press, 1982. [You read it correctly: *Pluto's Republic* – a good book about the mechanisms of discovery.]

Medvei, V. C., *A History of Endocrinology*, MTP Press, Hingham, Massachusetts, 1982. [Medvei openly admits that this compendium is an effort to update Rolleston's 1938 classic. Wonderful reading.]

Meites, J., *et al, Pioneers in Neuroendocrinology*, Plenum Press, New York, 1975. [In this slim volume, several of the great pioneers were encouraged to recall the 'incunabula' days of neuroendocrinology. Hinsey writes his story in detail in these pages.]

Melzack, R. and Wall, P. D., 'Pain Mechanisms; A New Theory', *Science*, 150, 971–9, 1965. [The first description of the 'gate control' theory of pain.]

Merril, C., *et al*, 'Regional Variations in Cerebrospinal Fluid Proteins', *Science*, 211, 1437–8, 1981. [As a preface to Merril's article, read P. H. O'Farrell's article in the *Journal of Biological Chemistry*, 250, 4007–21 written in 1975. In my discussions with clinicians I am surprised how few of them are aware of Merril's observations. If his observations obtain in humans, we have no choice but to measure hormones in the cerebral ventricles.]

Mettler, F., Personal communication. [Mettler and his wife co-authored an important text on the history of medicine in 1945. After her untimely death Mettler continued his medical sleuthing and has written, but not yet published, a book about John Hunter's dyslexia.]

Milhorat, T., 'The Third Circulation Revisited', *Journal of Neurosurgery*, 42, 628–45, 1975. [This article is the best on the question, 'Why is the brain hollow?']

Milhorat, T., 'Normal Rate of Cerebrospinal Formation after Bilateral Choroid Plexectomy', *Journal of Neurosurgery*, 44, 735–9, 1976. [The scientific evidence that choroid plexectomy is not effective in hydrocephalus is presented here.]

Milhorat, T., Mosher, M. B. and Hammock, M. K., 'Evidence for Choroid Plexus Absorption in Hydrocephalus', *New England Journal of Medicine*, 282, 286–9, 1970. [This gives the evidence that the choroid plexus removes labelled material from the ventricle; exactly the opposite of what Walter Dandy preached.]

Miller, N., 'Learning of Visceral and Glandular Responses', *Science*, 163, 434–45, 1969. [A western scientist confirms what has been eastern wisdom for centuries.]

Moniz, Egas, 'Essai d'un Traitement Chirurgical de Certaines Psychoses', *Bulletin de l'Académie de Medicine*, 115, 385–92, 1936. [In this, Moniz describes lobotomy for the first time. Later the Nobel committee would honor him, but most now regard this report as the beginning of a sad period in the history of neurosurgery. It is the best example of something that worked well in an 'electrically-based' laboratory, but failed miserably at the bedside.]

Montagu, M. F., *Studies and Essays in the History of Science*, Schuman, New York, 1945. [In 'The Bloodletting Letter of 1539', Vesalius's discontent with the doctrines of Galen are best expressed.]

Mostofi, B., Personal communication.

Nakane, P. K., 'Classification of Pituitary Cells by Immunohistochemistry', *Journal of Histochemistry and Cytochemistry*, 18, 9, 1970. [The first description of the horseradish peroxidase 'sandwich' that has become the workhorse for hormone localization in cells.]

Noda, M., *et al*, 'Cloning and Sequence Analysis of Adrenal Preproenkephalin', *Nature*, 295, 202–6, 1982. [This article describes 50–K – the giant prohormone in the adrenal which contains several linked enkephalin fragments.]

O'Malley, C. D. and Saunders, J. B., *Leonardo: On the Human Body*, Saunders, New York, 1952. [A beautiful book, but it shows that Leonardo was an artist, not a scientist.]

Ornstein, R. E., *The Psychology of Consciousness*, Freeman, New York, 1972. [Of all the popular books about the brain, I like this one the best, even though it is written by a 'soft' scientist.]

Osler, William, *The Evolution of Modern Medicine*, Yale University Press, New Haven, 1921. [This epic in scholarship shows why Osler, a professor of medicine, was Cushing's role model.]

Pare, Ambrose, *The Collected Works*, Milford House, New York, 1968. [This book contains descriptions of the ventricles that had to come from Galen. The illustrations of the ventricles are those of Vesalius.]

Pardridge, W., 'Brain Metabolism: A Perspective from the Blood Brain Barrier', *Physiological Reviews*, 63, 1481–535, 1983. [A review article which explains why the blood-brain barrier can no longer be thought of as a 'lead shield'; it is dynamic. Although Pardridge doesn't say so, the article leads me to think that many hormonally-related diseases of the brain come from disorders of the blood-brain barrier, not the brain itself.]

Paton, J. and Nottebohm, F., 'Neurones Generated in the Adult Brain are Recruited into Functional Circuits', *Science*, 225, 1046–8, 1984. [This

article shows that adult animals can produce new nerve cells; it challenges all that is 'holy' in neuroanatomy, especially the notion that each
of us suffers an irreplaceable loss of several million nerve cells each
day.]

Paton, W., 'The Action of Morphine ... on Guinea Pig Ileum', *British
Journal of Pharmacology and Chemotherapy*, 12, 119, 1957. [The
first description of the bio-assay that scientists use routinely to check
for 'opiate-like' activity; it was this test that allowed Hughes and
Kosterlitz to discover enkephalin.]

Pearse, A. G. E., 'Common Characteristics of Cells Producing Polypep-
tide Hormones', *Proceedings of the Royal Society of London*, 170, 71,
1968. [A description of the APUD system of hormone producing cells
that is scattered throughout the body. It permeates paracrinology.]

Peterson, O. H., *The Electrophysiology of Gland Cells*, Academic Press,
New York, 1980.

Pickering, G., *Creative Malady*, Allan and Unwin, London, 1974. [Read
this if you doubt that the best kind of lateral thinking is the conversion
of problems into opportunities.]

Plato, 'The Apology of Socrates and the Death of Socrates', in *World
Masterpieces*, Norton, New York, 1974. [In the *Apology*, Socrates's
penchant for questions is described; in the trial that led to his death are
warnings for all of those who find themselves asking questions about
new things instead of reciting answers about old things.]

Popa, G. T. and Fielding, U., 'A Portal Circulation from the Pituitary to
the Hypothalamic Region', *Journal of Anatomy*, 65, 88–91, 1930. [In
this, the first description of the pituitary portal system, it was clearly
stated that blood may flow from the pituitary to the brain. Although
most scientists since Wislocki have discounted this view, I believe it is
correct.]

Popper, K., *The Logic of Scientific Discovery*, Hutchinson; London, 1972.
[In this book Popper points out the subtle differences between scientific 'truths' and 'falsifications'.]

Potts, M., Short, R. and Best, W., 'The Thread of Life', [An informal
prospectus for a television program.] *Family Health International*,
Research Triangle Park, NC, 1983. [My statement, 'As our island of
knowledge grows, our shoreline of wonder should expand', came from
this.]

Ramon y Cajal, S. *Texture del sisteme nervioso del hombre y de los verte-
brados*, Moya, Madrid, 1899–1904. [In these publications, the synaptic
relationships between nerve cells are described for the first time.]

Rapoport, S. I., *Blood Brain Barrier in Physiology and Medicine*, Raven
Press, New York, 1976. [This is a lucid description of all aspects of the
blood brain barrier.]

Reti, L., *The Unknown Leonardo*, Hutchinson, London, 1974. [This
makes it clear that Leonardo's mirror-written words were notes to
himself.]

Reynolds, D. V., 'Surgery in the Rat during Electrical Anaesthesia',
Science, 164, 444–5, 1969. [The first description of analgesia after
electrical stimulation of the mid-brain. The studies of Akil and Hosobu-
chi come from this work.]

Rodgriquez, E. M., *et al.*, 'Neuroendocrine Mechanisms', *Frontiers of Hormone Research; Cerebrospinal Fluid and Peptide Hormones*, Karger, Basel, 142–58, 1980. [A description of the paradoxical ADH effect: rats were given anti-diuretic hormone into the ventricle and *lost water* instead of retaining it. The Dandy paradigm would predict that ADH placed into the ventricle would be carried first out of the brain and then into the blood stream. This article shows that doesn't happen.]

Rogers, G. *Brother Surgeons*, Dymock's, Sydney, 1957. [This book describes the differences between two brothers: John and William Hunter. William, the elder, had all the qualities of someone who is left-brain dominant while John, a dyslexic, was clearly driven by his right brain.]

Rolleston, H. D., *The Endocrine Organs in Health and Disease*, Oxford University Press, 1936. [This hard-to-get book is scholarship at its best. This was the model for my book.]

Rose, S., *The Conscious Brain*, Weidenfeld and Nicolson, London, 1973. [If Ornstein's book is the best book written by a 'soft' scientist about the brain, this is the best popular book written by a 'hard' scientist.]

Roth, J., *et al.*, 'The Evolutionary Origins of Hormones', *New England Journal of Medicine*, 306, 523, 1982. [To summarize this article: every hormone can be made everywhere and, it would seem, by every kind of creature.]

Rosenstein, J. and Brightman, M., 'Intact Cerebral Ventricle as a site for Tissue Transplantation', *Nature*, 275, 83–5, 1979. [An early and important article about brain transplantation.]

Russell, Bertrand, *A History of Western Philosophy*, London, 1946. [A well-written, well-illustrated classic containing the best description of the Platonic bodies I have read.]

Sartan, G., *Galen of Pergamon*, University of Kansas Press, Lawrence, 1954. [This book outlines the chicanery of Galen and his mid-life switch from 'scientist' to 'writer'. Reading it makes me believe many will compare my similar switch to Galen's.]

Scharrer, E. and Scharrer, B., *Neuroendocrinology*, Columbia University Press, New York, 1963. [The Scharrers, a husband and wife scientific team, outline in this book the fundamental principles of neuroendocrinology.]

Schleiden, M. J., 'Beitrage zur Phytogenesis', Muller's Archives, 1838. [This is the first description of *plant* cells.]

Schrodinger, E., *What is Life?*, Cambridge University Press, Cambridge, 1967. [This famous book contains the theoretical 'cat in a box' experiment which links the stuff of thought to the stuff of matter.]

Schwann, T., 'Microscopical Research on the Similarity in Structure and Growth of Animals and Plants', Muller's Archives, 1839. [The first description of *animal* cells.]

Seelig, K., *Albert Einstein*, Europa Verlag, Zurich, 1954. [From this, one important Einstein quote: 'I maintain that cosmic religiousness is the strongest and most noble driving force of scientific research. Only the man [*sic*] who can conceive the gigantic effort and above all the devotion, without which original scientific thought cannot succeed, can measure the strength of feeling from which alone such work ... can grow. What a deep belief in the intelligence of Creation and what long-ing for understanding, even if only of a meagre reflection in the revealed intelligence of this world, must have flourished in Kepler and Newton, enabling them as lonely men to unravel over years of work the mechanism of celestial mechanics... Only the man [*sic*] who devotes his life to such goals has a living conception of what inspired these men and gave them strength to remain steadfast in their aims in spite of count-less failures. It is cosmic religiousness that bestows such strength. A contemporary has said, not unrightly, that the serious research scholar in our generally materialistic age is the only deeply religious human being.']

Selverstone, B., 'Studies of Cerebrospinal Fluid [in humans] using Radio-active Tracers', *Ciba Symposium*, London, 147–67, 1958. [In this, Selverstone shows that a radioactive tracer placed in the ventricle is found almost instantly in the bloodstream but does not appear in the cisterna for fifteen minutes. This is incompatible with the Dandy para-digm for brain water.]

Shealy, N., *et al.*, 'Dorsal Column Electroanalgesia', *Journal of Neuro-surgery*, 32, 560–4, 1970. [The first description of a space-age techni-que that was the outgrowth of the 'gate control' theory.]

Sherrington, C., *The Integrative Action of the Nervous System*, Yale University Press, New Haven, 1906. [Here Sherrington sets in place the essentials of the 'hard-wired' view of an electrically driven brain.]

Siegel, R. E., *Galen's System of Physiology and Medicine*, Karger, Basel, 1968.

Singer, C., *Galen on Anatomical Procedures*, Oxford University Press, London, 1956, and *From Magic to Science*, Benn, London, 1928. [Both contain descriptions of Galen's prodigious works and writings.]

Sperry, R. W., 'Perception in the Absence of Neocortical Commissures', in *Perception and its Disorders*, The Annual Research Publication of the Association for Research in Nervous and Mental Disease, Vol. 48, 1970. [As Sperry taught us, we have two brains: a 'savant' on the left who reads and writes and a 'mystic' on the right, imbued with *a priori* knowledge, who dreams.]

Spiller, W. G. and Frazier, C. H., 'The Division of the Sensory Root of the Trigeminus for the Relief of Tic Douloureaux, *Philadelphia Medical Journal*, 8, 1039–49, 1901. [All surgical procedures which divide nerves in the name of pain relief grow from this publication.]

Strand, F., 'Endocrineurology', in *Humoral Control of Growth and Differentiation*, Academic Press, 1973. [Many will quarrel with my separation of 'neuroendocrinology' and 'endocrine neurology'. Fleur Strand said so first.]

Swaab, D. F., 'Neuropeptides: Their Distribution in the Brain', *Progress in Brain Research*, 55, 97–122, 1982. [The title contains the summary, yet in this rapidly changing field even this recent article is now out of date.]

Sweet, W. H. and Wepsic, J. G., 'Treatment of Pain by (percutaneous) Stimulation?', *Transactions of the American Neurological Associa-tion*, 93, 103–7, 1968. [It was this observation that led to the use of percutaneous nerve stimulation in the treatment of pain. Sweet knows more about pain than anyone I know and supports the notion that we will treat it effectively only when we know more about brain endocrinology.]

Tache, Y., *et al.*, 'CNS Mediated Inhibition of Gastric Secretion by Bombesin', *Regulatory Peptides*, 3, 105–12, 1982. [Bombesin, which was first found in frog skin, mysteriously quietens the activity of the stomach. This only occurs, however, if it is placed in the ventricle. Again this demonstrates why the ventricle is important to hormonal therapy of the brain.]

Tanaka, I. *et al.*, 'Presence of ... (31–K) ... Peptides in Human Stomach', *Journal of Clinical and Endocrinological Metabolism*, 54, 392–6 1982. [Link this to the article of Kruseman which shows CRF, which releases 31–K, in the gut. Then ask, 'Can the gut think?']

Tower, D. (ed.), *The Nervous System* [3 vols], Raven Press, New York, 1975. [In the year these volumes were published, enkephalin was found in the brain. Looking back at the articles now, less than a decade later, most of them seem out of date for there is nothing about brain hormones.]

Tsong, S. D., *et al.*, 'ACTH and Endorphin are Present in Multiple Sites of the Reproductive Tract', *Endocrinology*, 110, 2204–6, 1982. [The articles of Kruseman and Tanaka make me wonder if the gut can think. Wathes describes ovarian vasopressin, which also releases 31–K. This makes me ask, 'Can the ovaries think?']

Vale, W., *et al.*, 'The Characterization of Corticotropin Releasing Factor', *Science*, 213, 1394–7, 1981. [For nearly thirty years scientists searched for this substance, now called CRF. This has been described as the 'holy grail' of neuroendocrinology. Wylie Vale, the leader of the team that found it, had earlier worked with Roger Guillemin on TRF.]

Vesalius, Andreas, *De Humanis Corporis Fabricus*, Basel, 1543. [This book is the Veda, Torah, Bible and Koran of medicine; its very birthright. There are many good reproductions of it in bookstores which deserve examination. Remarkably, the original editions were printed on such good paper that they remain in excellent condition. Harvard's Countway Library has seven first editions of the *Fabric of Man*; they are protected, but available for examination.]

Virchow, R., *Cellular Pathology*, Berlin, 1858. [Virchow is the pathologist who best articulated the 'cellular theory', yet he held on to Schwann's mismeme of the 'network theory' of brain function.]

Von Neumann, J., *The Computer and the Brain*, Yale University Press, New Haven, Connecticutt, 1958. [The title articulates a widely held comparison, still honoured in most academic bastions. This simplistic comparison I eschew: the brain is more like a gland than a computer.]

Wade, N. and Broad, W., *Betrayers of the Truth*, Simon and Schuster, New York, 1983. [Tales of 'falsifications' in the laboratory, some of which I have seen first hand.]

Wathes, D. C., *et al.*, 'Neurohypophyseal Hormones in Human Ovary', *Lancet*, 2, 410–12, 1982. [Link this to Tsong's article to know that the combination of molecules that the brain employs to 'think' is found in the ovary.]

Watson, J. D. and Crick, F. H. C., 'Molecular Structure of Nucleic Acids', *Nature*, 171, 737–8, 1953. [In Medawar's book, *Pluto's Republic*, this one-page publication is described as the most important scientific paper of the twentieth century.]

Weed, L. H., 'The Absorption of Cerebrospinal Fluid into the Venous System', *American Journal of Anatomy*, 31, 191–221, 1923. [This is a description of the 'Paccionnian' granulations through which some CSF enters the bloodstream.]

Weiner, J., *Cybernetics*, Wiley, New York, 1948. [The term 'cybernetics', comes from the Greek word for helmsman. The notion that reverberating, cybernetic electrical currents serve as the helmsmen for the mind has been in vogue for several decades.]

Weiss, P. and Hiscoe, H. B., 'Experiments in the Mechanism of Nerve Growth', *Journal of Experimental Zoology*, 107, 315–93, 1948. [This was the first paper to talk about 'axoplasmic flow' – the movement of bulk material down nerve trunks.]

Wells, H. G., *Mankind in the Making*, Chapman and Hall, London, 1903. [It is clear to all historians, especially H. G. Wells, that the dark ages began during Galen's time.]

Whitehead, A. N., *Science and the Modern World*, Mentor, New York, 1948. [This classic stresses the importance of models for thought in new discoveries.]

Wilson, C., *Starseekers*, Hodder and Stoughton, London, 1980. [A splendid book about cosmology. It documents how long the mismeme of the Platonic bodies existed: Kepler in AD 1595 concluded that the relationships between planets corresponded to the relationships of the five Platonic bodies.]

Wislocki, G. B. and King, L. S., 'A Study of the Hypophysial Vascular Supply', *American Journal of Anatomy*, 58, 421–72, 1936. [This is the classic description of the 'pituitary portal system'.]

Wright, R. D., 'What Australian Physiology Owes to Adolph Hitler', *Proceedings of the Australian Physiological Society*, 14, 22–7, 1983. [Sir Douglas Wright writes here about Feldberg's 'transfer' from England to Australia.]

Yates, F. E., *et al.*, 'Potentiation by Vasopressin of Corticotropin Release Induced by Corticotropin-Releasing Factor', *Endocrinology*, 88, 3–15, 1971. [This is the first of the many articles which confirm that ADH and CRF come together as a 'hormonal harmony' to trigger the release of 31–K. My most recent work in the laboratory has focused on this curious synergism; plasma endorphin elevations have been observed repeatedly in sheep that were given ADH and CRF.]

Numbers in italics indicate illustrations.